A Beginners Guid
Bach Flower Remedies

Bach Flower remedies are natural medicines made from
flowers. They have the power to resolve the negative and
spiritual states that are the root cause of disease. This
introductory guide is designed to help you start using the
remedies for yourself, and includes:

- the nature and history of the remedies
- case histories showing how the remedies work
- how to select and take the right remedies
- how to find good practitioners

Contents

INTRODUCTION

BEFORE WE START

'Bach' is pronounced 'Batch', to rhyme with 'match'. Now that we have got that question out of the way, we can move on...

WESTERN MEDICINE

The Western world's approach to dealing with health has on the whole been extremely successful. So much so that even countries like India and China, which have their own very different medical traditions, now accept and use the West's model.

But what exactly is orthodox, Western medicine?

At the risk of over simplifying we could say that Western medicine represents a reductionist, physical approach based on the use of drugs and technology. It is reductionist because it reduces people to sets of symptoms so as to intervene at that level. It is physical because it deals almost exclusively with bodies. And the fact that it is based on drugs and technology is graphically shown by the different values placed on people and machines in most modern health services: money is lavished on new drugs and new machines, while nurses are paid a pittance.

If you have a wheeze in your chest the doctor will start by listening to your breathing. Then he will prescribe a drug or other treatment designed to deal with the inflammation or congestion or whatever that is causing the wheeze. If the doctor does ask you how you feel apart from the wheeze you will probably understand this to relate to your physical condition. You are likely to mention a sore throat; less likely to mention the fact that you lost your job yesterday.

This approach is very effective at dealing with physical symptoms like the wheezing chest, because drugs are tailor made to attack the physical cause of the illness. It is also spectacularly successful when it comes to injuries such as fractured legs, ribs and skulls. The doctor can use the technological equipment at her disposal to isolate the problem, and then use physical means to repair it - straightening the leg, binding up the rib and tacking metal plates onto the skull. Lives are saved every day using scientific Western medicine.
But for many it is still failing.

PEOPLE AS CARS

The magic bullet idea of medicine - that there is a physical solution to every physical symptom - is in turn based on a philosophical view of human life that stresses the complete separateness of our physical and mental worlds. 'I think therefore I am' said Descartes, but the 'I' he was talking about was not his stomach or his arms or his heart. Instead 'I' is somewhere up here in the head. 'I' looks out through its eyes, and its body is something else, a sort of vehicle that 'I' uses to get carried around in. The thoughts and feelings of 'I' don't have any real effect on the body because there is no direct connection. 'I' can do what it wants with its body, as long as it gets it serviced from time to time and takes on enough fuel.

Perhaps this explains why some of us treat our bodies much the same as we treat our cars: we go too fast; we don't look after ourselves; we crash; we take ourselves off to the doctor to be fixed up. Doctors become glorified garage mechanics, replacing worn out parts and rebuilding bits of broken machinery.

A PROBLEM WITH THE ORTHODOX APPROACH

To continue the metaphor, one problem with the orthodox approach is that while the car is being repaired the driver is often not treated at all. He sits around waiting for the vehicle to be fixed, then off he goes, driving just as badly as before, until once again he crashes.

The main criticism of the orthodox approach is that it does not do enough for that part of us that cannot be seen. The 'I' in its head is not considered, when in fact the 'I' is often the cause of the body's problem. And beyond the 'I', at the level of spirit or soul, the problem is worse. For modem Western medicine the soul of the patient is not only not considered: for all practical reasons it isn't even there at all.

HOLISTIC MEDICINE

Dr Bach once gave a simple instruction to his team: 'treat the person, not the disease.' This is the holistic approach in a nutshell.

Holism puts forward the view that spirit, mind and body are interconnected in countless subtle ways. Holistic medicine seeks to view and treat people in their entirety so as to address all aspects of our lives at once.

Some methods, such as reflexology and acupuncture, direct the majority of their attention at physical problems, but do so using a system that also affects the mental and spiritual side of our beings. Others take a mixed approach and seek to prescribe for both levels at once - homoeopathy would be a good example of this, with its mix of physical and mental symptomatology.

With Bach Flower Remedies, however, diagnosis is purely on the level of spirit and mind, on the theory that balances at this level will in turn affect the health of the body. 'Take no notice of the disease,' wrote Dr Bach, 'think only of the outlook on life of the one in distress.' Emotional states are used as the key to unlock the body's natural health.

PSYCHONEUROIMMUNOLOGY

In many ways the holistic argument is becoming part of the mainstream. Most doctors now accept that stress and emotional imbalance contribute to anything up to 95%of all disease, and there has been a flurry of research in the United States into the effect of emotions on the immune system. Dr Robert Ader, working on this subject at the University of Rochester in 1975, was the first person to call this subject psychoneuroimmunology, or PNI for short.

PNI is the study of how people's states of mind influence their physical health through links between the brain and the immune system. At first a fringe activity, more and more mainstream scientists now work in this area. Positive research results have appeared in major professional journals such as the UK journal The Lancet and the US Proceedings of the National Academy of Sciences. It has been demonstrated that stress leads to the release of neurotransmitters and hormones, and that these in turn change cellular activity in the immune system. It seems that the immune system is equipped with receptors that can receive emotional messages from the brain.

An article in the US journal The Scientist mentions important work in this area. At Ohio State University, for example, one study found that people struggling with the pressures of caring for relatives with Alzheimer's disease tended to suffer from worse colds than other people. Another showed that people with high anxiety levels had less effective protection from antibodies and immune cells.

PNI tends to confirm what holism has always claimed, that a lack of harmony in the mental or spiritual area will lead eventually to physical illness. And a further interesting result of PNI research has been to show that people who feel in control of their lives and emotions are less likely to be sick than those who feel that they are controlled by fate, the elements, or some other external force.

WHAT ARE BACH FLOWER REMEDIES?

This is where Bach Flower Remedies fit in. They are medicines for the emotions, which aim to balance negative states of mind and resolve character defects by encouraging the corresponding virtue. This means that we can all gain the health benefits of having a balanced emotional life. And because they are simple tools that anyone can learn to use, they give us all the power to take control of our emotional lives. We can all be inner-directed, and as PNI research has shown, this alone can lead us to feel healthier and better about our lives.

There are 38 basic remedies in the system. 37 of them are made from a single flower or plant; one is especially prepared spring water. Each remedy is aimed at a specific negative emotion, such as fear, lack of confidence or worry; and the result of taking the remedy is to give courage, increase confidence and quiet the worrying mind.

The remedies do not work in the same way that orthodox drugs would, by dampening down symptoms. Instead they work by enhancing our existing positive qualities. The negative state isn't suppressed, but removed by an increase in the corresponding positive quality.

Bach Flower Remedies bring holistic healing into the hands of everyone. That is why Or Bach was fond of referring to them as the medicine of the future. Before growing towards that future, however, it will be helpful to look back at the roots of the system, and to answer the obvious question: 'Who was this Dr Bach, and where did these remedies come from?'

CHAPTER 1

WHERE DO BACH FLOWER REMEDIES COME FROM?

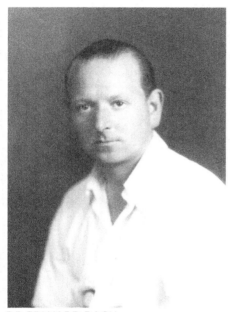

DR EDWARD BACH

The man who discovered the 38 remedies was called Edward Bach. He was born in the West Midlands in 1886, where his father owned a brass foundry. When he left school he worked at
the foundry for a time, but he felt a calling towards healing and soon left to study medicine, first at Birmingham University and later at University College Hospital in London, where he qualified in 1912.

Trained as an orthodox doctor, Bach's career path started off in an equally orthodox manner. After qualifying he took a place as Casualty Medical Officer at University College Hospital, and he also held the post of Casualty House Surgeon at the National Temperance Hospital until his own ill health obliged him to give up that position. He opened his own consulting rooms near Harley Street, and soon became interested in immunology, leading to research work as a bacteriologist at University College Hospital.

It was here that he first began to make a name for himself as an original thinker. He was intrigued by the problem of chronic disease, and by its possible relationship to certain bacteria that seemed to proliferate in the intestines of patients. He produced seven vaccines from the seven different types of bacteria he found, and gave them to his patients. The results were extremely good.

When the First World War started in 1914Bach tried to enlist, but was turned down repeatedly because of his poor state of health. Determined to do what he could, he took on extra duties at the hospital, where he was in charge of more than 400 beds reserved for war casualties. His research work continued unabated, while his health deteriorated to such a degree that in 1917he suffered a haemorrhage and lost consciousness.

An immediate operation was carried out to remove a cancerous growth; but the prognosis was poor, and when Bach came round his colleagues told him that at the very most he had three months left to live.

Bach left his hospital bed as soon as he was able to walk, and plunged himself back into his work. If he only had a little time, then he would use it to make as great a contribution as he could, and complete if possible his work on chronic disease.

He worked every hour of the day and night. He was so wrapped up in his research and war work that he hardly noticed that his strength was returning and that he had already outlived the most optimistic of his colleagues' predictions. In her biography, Nora Weeks tells of one of the doctors who had treated Bach returning from the front some time after the operation. He was so surprised to see Bach walking around that he greeted him with the words: 'But, good God! Bach, you're dead!'

Ever since his days in the brass foundry Bach had been aware that the fear of illness was as great a problem as the illness itself. Workers were terrified of falling ill because it would mean the loss of income and so no food on the table; and the fear alone seemed to make illness more likely. Thinking now about his own miraculous recovery he saw a link between his reaction to the diagnosis of cancer and his return to health. He became convinced that he had got better because he was too engaged with life and with his life's work to feel fear. His vocation had saved him.

HOMOEOPATHIC PRINCIPLES

Bach's work with the bacterial vaccines was very successful, but there were some aspects of it that he found distasteful. In particular he disliked the idea of giving injections to patients. He found a partial answer to this problem when he found that he got better results by only giving further doses of the vaccine once all improvement from the first dose had stopped. Instead of giving injections at regular intervals the new method meant that sometimes he only had to give a repeat dose after many months.

The next big breakthrough came in 1919, when Bach started work as a pathologist and bacteriologist at the London Homoeopathic Hospital. Required reading for this new job was Samuel Hahnemann's seminal work The Organon of Rational

Medicine. As he read the book Bach was startled to find that without knowing it he had been following in Hahnemann's footsteps: the founder of homoeopathy had identified the principle of the minimum dose and the link between intestinal toxaemia and chronic disease a century before. Bach also felt great sympathy with the homoeopathic principle of treating people as individuals rather than concentrating on the disease alone; and with the use in some homoeopathic remedies of natural plants.

THE SEVEN BACH NOSODES

It was natural for Bach to wonder how other ideas contained in the Organon might relate to his own work. Accordingly, he tried preparing his vaccines using homoeopathic methods. The results were excellent, and as the homoeopathic vaccines were administered by mouth he was able to abandon the use of injections. The new homoeopathic vaccines became known as the seven Bach nosodes. They are still in use today.

TREATING THE PERSON, NOT THE DISEASE

Homoeopathic medicines are not only prescribed for the patient's physical symptoms. Practitioners also take account of the type of person being treated and of her state of mind. These non-physical symptoms are often referred to as 'mentals'.

Bach began to make notes on the different personalities of the people he was treating. Soon he was able to build up a picture of the mentals associated with each of the seven nosodes. As time went by he found he was able to predict which nosode a person needed from observation of his character alone. He still used laboratory analysis of bacterial specimens, but more and more this was only to confirm a diagnosis already arrived at.

Despite these successes he remained less than satisfied with what he had achieved. He was making the nosodes from bacteria taken from the intestines of sick people. The nosodes were the products of disease. He disliked the idea of building health on sickness, and was convinced that somewhere in nature there would be a purer type of medicine that would be wholly positive in its action.

THE THEORY OF TYPES

Dr Bach began to collect plants and take them back to his laboratories. There he prepared and tested them using standard homoeopathic methods, and compared the resulting medicine with his original nosodes. Over time he found some plants that had a similar effect to the nosodes, but the match was never exact.

One night Bach was attending an official dinner. Out of boredom he began to observe the other guests, and it came to him in a flash that all the people there could be divided into groups, according to their characters and behaviour, and in much the same way that he divided people into groups when selecting a nosode for them.

However, instead of only seven groups he quickly sketched out more. He wondered at first whether each of these new groups would be associated with a particular disease, but he quickly realised that this was not so. Rather, each group of people would tend to react in the same ways to any disease that they caught.

Up to this point Bach's work had only been aimed at a specific kind of chronic disease. Now he saw how the new scheme that he had begun to sketch out might lead to a truly complete system, one which would be able to treat all diseases. It would do this by treating people's basic emotional imbalances directly.

This would represent a much greater application of the homoeopathic principle of treating the whole person than any seen so far.

DISCOVERY OF THE FLOWER REMEDIES

In September 1928 Dr Bach found the first of the plants that were to form part of the system of 38 flower remedies. These were Impatiens and Mimulus, which he brought back to London from Wales, and prepared in his laboratory in the same way as he had prepared so many plants before.

He matched the plants to two of the personality groups that he had worked out, and tried them on his patients. A third remedy was soon added to the first two, this time made from Clematis.

The results were so good that by the end of the following year Bach had stopped using the nosodes completely. A few months later, early in 1930, he decided to leave London so as to devote himself full-time to finding more healing plants and to the development of the new system. His colleagues were stunned by his decision, but his conviction and enthusiasm were such that Bach overcame all objections. By May of that year he was on his way, accompanied by his assistant Nora Weeks, who had agreed to go with him.

Bach spent the next four years travelling all over the southern half of Britain, from Wales to East Anglia. He walked much of the time, constantly looking for new plants to prepare; but the first discovery he made was of a new method of preparing remedies, one that was far simpler than any in homoeopathy, and one more in keeping with his wish to find a natural medicine.

THE SUN METHOD

Even before he left London Bach was aware that his sensitivity towards the energy in plants had been growing. He was able to feel the effects of a flower simply by holding it in his hands: some would bring calm and strength, while others would cause nausea and other physical reactions.

Bach discovered his new method of capturing the potency of these flowers very early one sunny morning, when he was walking through a field in Wales. The flowers around about were covered in dew. It occurred to him that the heat of the sun might be enough to draw the potency in the flowers into the liquid, so creating a natural preparation.

He decided to test out this theory, and set to work to collect the dewdrops. Some he took from flowers that had been in full sunlight, and others from plants growing in the shade. The results confirmed his intuition: there was indeed a potency in the liquid he had collected, and it was far stronger in the dew taken from the sun-warmed flowers.

The next step was to find a practical way of using this discovery.

It would take too long to collect dew from flowers, so Bach tried using a bowl of water instead. He collected flowers and laid them on the bowl in the sunlight. After a time he tested the resulting liquid, and to his delight it was as strong as the dew had been.

This method was the one that he used to prepare all of the remedies he found during his period of wandering – nineteen of them in all.

MOUNT VERNON

By 1934, Dr Bach was looking for somewhere more permanent to live. He had always liked the Thames valley, so when Nora Weeks found a small empty cottage called Mount Vernon available for rent in Sotwell, just outside Wallingford, he decided to take it. Having done so, he was delighted to find that most of the nineteen remedies he had already discovered grew in the countryside around his new house.

Funds were low - Bach spent all he had on his work, and rarely charged for help - so he built much of the furniture for the house himself. He also threw himself into the garden, digging out the worst of the weeds and planting wild flowers by throwing handfuls of seeds into the air. In more orthodox garden fashion, he also laid out some small lawns and used some of the rubble left around to layout paths.

THE LAST NINETEEN REMEDIES

Dr Bach had nineteen remedies already - but he was aware that there were gaps in the system, and in the spring of 1935 he again began to look for new remedies.

His sensitivity at this time had developed to an alarming degree, and he began to suffer intensely from the negative states of mind for which he needed remedies. Often a negative emotional state would be accompanied by severe physical pain; nevertheless he would go out and look for the plant that he needed to rebalance his emotions. At this time he really was his own laboratory.

He suffered in this way all through the spring and summer of 1935. By August he had found a further nineteen remedies. The system was complete: he now had a remedy for every basic negative emotion that people could suffer.

THE BOILING METHOD

The first of the new series of remedies was found in March. At this time Dr Bach was suffering from a severe sinusitis, which was accompanied by a feeling of utter desperation, as though he was losing his mind. He wanted to prepare the blossoming twigs of the Cherry Plum tree, which his intuition told him might be the cure he sought. But in March the sun was not warm enough to potentise such tough plant material using the sun method, so Dr Bach needed to look for a different means of extracting the healing essence.

He decided to try boiling up the flowering twigs in water to see if this would be as effective. This he did, boiling them for a time and then allowing the pan to cool and filtering off the liquid. He took a few drops of the liquid, and the desperation and pain faded at once, confirming the choice of plant and the usefulness of this new method of preparation.

THE BACH CENTRE

Edward Bach died on November 27th 1936, over a year after completing his work and writing up his findings. He left all he had to Nora Weeks, and in particular he asked her and Victor Bullen, another close friend who had helped him for many years, to continue his work following the principles he had set out. 'As soon as a teacher has given his work to the world, a contorted version of the same must arise,' he wrote to Victor a month before his death. 'Our work is steadfastly to adhere to the simplicity and purity of this method of healing.'

Nora and Victor saw out the difficult years of the Second World War, making remedies every year, and giving consultations and advice to the many people who arrived at the house looking for help. Over the years news of the remedies spread.

They were never advertised: word of mouth and personal recommendation was enough for them to spread, little by little, all over the world.

Supporters of their work raised the money to allow them to buy Mount Vernon in 1958, and Nora and Victor set up a trust so that the house and garden would remain the centre of Dr Bach's work for all time, as he had intended. Over the years the house and the people in it became known as the Bach Centre.

Victor died in 1975, Nora three years later. But they had already made plans to pass on responsibility for the work to John Ramsell and his sister Nickie Murray. Nickie decided to retire in 1988, and John's daughter Judy Howard took her place as a trustee. Both are still there today, along with a small team of five other people.

Up until 1991 the remedies were still bottled and packed and sent out from Mount Vernon. One small outbuilding housed the world distribution centre. But in 1991 the business of getting remedies to 66 countries and millions of people all over the world was transferred to the homoeopathic company A Nelson & Co.

This left the Bach Centre time and space in which to resume one part of Dr Bach's work that had never been completed. Back in 1936, on his birthday, Dr Bach had given an address in Wallingford in the first of a planned series of lectures, aimed at spreading news of his discoveries to as many people as possible. In 1991 the old bottling centre at Mount Vernon was converted into a seminar room, and the first of a series of courses was held, aimed at training professional practitioners to use the remedies in the simple way that Dr Bach used them.

Like the remedies, Bach Centre-approved courses are now available in many different countries around the world, and the register of trained practitioners held at the Centre grows by more than 25% every year.

This work sits well alongside the continuing commitment at the Centre to free help and advice, and, in the spring and summer, with the Centre's continuing role in the most important activity of all: making the remedies.

CHAPTER 2

WHO USES BACH FLOWER REMEDIES?

ON SIMPLICITY

At the end of so many years of research into so many different aspects of medicine, you might have expected that Dr Bach would leave behind him shelves full of massive textbooks, complete with footnotes and appendices, and understandable only after long study and a great deal of effort.

In fact he summed up his life's work in about 30 pages, in a little booklet called The Twelve Healers and Other Remedies. And throughout his life he destroyed his notes and all evidence of the work that had gone into creating the system of 38 remedies: he burned in a bonfire at Mount Vernon much of the material that might have ended up making the bookshelves groan.

He was clear about the reason for doing this. He wanted to avoid leaving behind anything that might complicate the system and make it harder for ordinary people to use. This wish comes across clearly in the introduction to the final version of The Twelve Healers:

This system of treatment is the most perfect which has been given to mankind within living memory. It has the power to cure disease; and, in its simplicity, it may be used in the household.

It is its simplicity, combined with its all-healing effects, that is so wonderful.

No science, no knowledge is necessary, apart from the simple methods described herein; and they who will obtain the greatest benefit from this God-sent gift will be those who keep it pure as it is; free from science, free from theories, for everything in Nature is simple.

Simplicity was one of Dr Bach's favourite words. It was the cornerstone of his approach to medicine, an approach that people today call empowerment. Thanks to empowerment the patient does not have to remain patient. Instead she is able to grasp the system herself, and use it to heal her own illnesses.

Over the years many people have come up with new ways of using the remedies, new approaches to selection and dosage, and new theories as to how they work. But the simple system that Dr Bach discovered remains what it has always been: the most effective system for self-help and self-healing ever discovered, the easiest to learn, and the simplest to use.

SELF-HEALING

During the decades that have passed since Dr Bach made his discoveries, most of the people who have used the remedies have used them for self-help. Sometimes self-help means a straightforward application of Rescue Remedy or Rescue Cream, at other times it means dealing with quite complex problems that require many different mixes of remedies. Here are some examples.

NORMAN'S STORY

'I am 78 and in good health. Recently a small growth developed on the bridge of my nose that would not heal. My doctor referred me to the dermatologist at the hospital. After examination and consultation with a surgeon the specialist said the only effective remedy would be to remove the growth by surgery under local anaesthetic, for which I should await an appointment.

To prevent occasional bleeding I subsequently covered the growth with a dressing on which it occurred to me to apply some Rescue Cream which had been unused in my medicine cupboard for some years.

Two days later the growth disappeared leaving no sign or scar on my skin.'

BEATRICE'S STORY

'I suffer from multiple sclerosis, and frequently suffer extreme exhaustion of my muscles. Such was the case recently when I had a lot of planting to do in the garden. I decided to take some Olive.

'After half an hour nothing seemed to be happening and so I felt that I must press on regardless. I completed the work that had to be done - it took about three hours – and suddenly I realised that I was not tired at all.

'I initially expected to get a sudden surge of energy after taking the Olive. Now I realise it doesn't work like that. I got on with the work and the tiredness just wasn't there anymore.'

CLAIRE'S STORY

'Recently I had to go into hospital for major surgery, and was very apprehensive as I dread pain. From the day I knew my admission date I took Water Violet (my type remedy), with Mimulus for my specific fears and Rescue Remedy.

'I found this significantly reduced my apprehension, so that I faced the ordeal calmly and with happiness that it would soon be over, rather than dreading its approach. I am glad to say that

I came through, feeling that my fear of pain had been unfounded and that the most I had suffered in that way was minor discomfort.'

JOSHUA'S STORY

'I come from a family with numerous mental and emotional disorders. In my early teens I began having episodes of deep depression, like a dark, gloomy cloud that came out of nowhere and parked itself over my head. By the time I was 20 I decided that allopathic medicine had only drugs to offer, so I determined to find my own answers.

'Homoeopathic treatment, acupuncture and herbs all helped to some degree, but despite all attempts the thread of the depression persisted.

Then I bought a set of Bach Flower Remedies and a book on how to use them. The description of Mustard fitted my symptoms perfectly, so I began to take it. The periods of depression lessened and became further and further apart. I continued with this remedy for nine months, at which time I stopped taking it. The depression has not returned at all.'

SHEILA'S STORY

'My son was born by Caesarean section after a full day in labour. Although I had been greatly looking forward to having the baby I could not shake off feelings of depression, exhaustion, fear, and over-anxiety about the child. My mind was running riot with imaginary fears. I even had a few panic attacks, which I've never had before.

'After two months of this a friend dosed me with a mix of Bach Flower Remedies - I can't remember what they were - and at the same time I started taking iron tablets. The mental exhaustion went, and I put my recovery down to the extra iron.

'However, seven months after the birth I was still suffering from over-anxiety, irritability, feelings of not being able to get everything done, and a consequent fear of losing my temper. So I got some books on the remedies - The Twelve Healers, Questions and Answers and Bach Flower Remedies Step by Step - and from these I decided that I needed Cherry Plum, Hornbeam and Mimulus.

'I dosed myself day and night (the baby wakes for two or three feeds at night) and after two and a half weeks I began to feel more mellow. After three weeks I felt so much myself again that I felt no need to continue with the remedies. In fact I feel better than I used to - and I have an increased sense of enjoyment of my baby, instead of an over-anxious care.'

RAY'S STORY

'At the age of 21 I had a severe nervous breakdown, which left me incapable of communicating with the outside world. It meant that I could not go outside my house for nearly a year without anxiety attacks.

'The breakdown was brought on by pressure from my father who was a very wealthy and successful businessman. He tried to mould my character so that I would follow in his footsteps. My personality was being suppressed and I finally cracked.

'I was prescribed valium, which is no cure but is a temporary relief. My mother then contacted a top psychiatrist who was very understanding and helpful. After two months I came off the valium and tried to combat my fears with his help and advice alone. For ten years I slowly improved, but I had reached an emotional barrier: I could go out and meet people and do all the things needed to survive and work in this world, but I still got anxiety attacks.

'I tried homoeopathy, but after a year I was still at the barrier. I became depressed as I thought I had reached the limits of my recovery. I saw the prospect of living the rest of my life with irrational and uncontrollable anxiety.

'Then I discovered Bach Flower Remedies. After three months my life had changed so dramatically that even now I cannot believe it. The emotional barrier dropped and I felt free. It was fantastic - a new life.

'Up until my breakdown I had been an engineer, but during the ten years that followed I discovered creativity within myself and started writing music. Now I am acting under a professional name, and appeared recently in a top TV soap series. You can imagine what an achievement that is for a man who once could not even walk out the front door.'

PRACTITIONERS

From time to time people using the remedies do get stuck, and when that happens they might go to see a professional practitioner. This might be someone who is using the remedies as one of many therapeutic approaches, or someone who specialises entirely in Bach Flower Remedies. In either case the results can repay the investment, as the following examples show.

NATALIE'S STORY

At her consultation Natalie sat on the edge of her chair and looked nervous, although she smiled all the time. She told the practitioner that she was feeling tense and anxious about forthcoming college examinations. She felt frightened of failing and of letting herself down, and of the effects a failure would have on her future plans. Yet at the same time she was finding it hard to get motivated enough to study, and kept finding reasons to put off looking at her books.

As the consultation went on she seemed to be uncomfortable with having to talk about herself, although she continued to smile and laugh at every opportunity. She said she was a confident person on the whole, and expected to succeed. However, she had taken on a lot recently - as well as her college work she was holding down a parttime job in a supermarket and learning to drive - and she was feeling more under pressure than usual, which perhaps accounted for her lack of confidence about the exams.

The way Natalie presented herself during the consultation, wearing a smile even as she was describing how anxious she felt, was a clear indication for Agrimony. Larch was the first choice for the lack of confidence and fear of failure, but when this remedy was explained to Natalie she made it clear that she felt she was a confident person – and it was true that she had not hesitated to take on a large number of commitments. When she heard the indications for Elm, however, she agreed at once that this described how she was feeling: a capable person who had taken on too much. Elm was given instead of Larch, and Mimulus was added because of her specific fears about her future if the exams did not go well.

Finally, Hornbeam was added to Natalie's mix so as to help her over her tendency to put off revising.

The exams went well; but the fall-out in other areas of her life was in some ways more interesting. As she took the remedies over a number of weeks she found that she became more comfortable with acknowledging and expressing the way she felt. On one occasion she talked through a problem with four friends, something which she would never have done before; and on another she was able to discuss a difficult situation with her mother and find a resolution, whereas before she would have pretended that all was well. People commented on how relaxed she seemed compared to her normal self, and wondered to what they should attribute the changes.

STEPHANIE'S STORY

Stephanie came for help because she was struggling with an unusually large workload, which was causing her a great deal of unhappiness and stress. She worked as a personal consultant, and as a board member of a prestigious professional organisation in her field she had landed the job of organising that organisation's next international convention. She was an efficient woman with a forceful personality, and used to organising other people, but she quickly found that this task took all her waking moments and brought her into conflict with other equally strong people. The job was all the more difficult because she was not getting any help or advice from the previous organiser, a fact that she resented. As the months went on she began to put on weight, and felt tired, frustrated and tense.

The main remedies that the practitioner selected for Stephanie were: Elm, for her feeling of being overwhelmed by the demands being made on her; Beech, to help her feel more tolerance for other people's views within the orgainisation; Mimulus, for the specific fears that she had of things going wrong; Willow, for her resentment over having been put in this situation; and Oak, because she was struggling on despite her exhaustion. White Chestnut was also given, to help overcome the obsessive, repetitive thoughts that kept her awake at night, and which were contributing to her tiredness.

As Stephanie said later on, as soon as she began taking these remedies she felt things beginning to move inside her, and instead of seeing her task as a looming nightmare she actually began to enjoy herself. By the time the actual convention came around she was a tower of strength, enthusiasm and diplomacy. Nobody who saw her in action could have guessed how negative she had felt only a few months before.

GORDON'S STORY

Gordon was 24 years old and single. For the past seven years he had been taking drugs for depression, but he remained full of fear and more recently had suffered some physical side-effects from the treatment. His doctor advised him to try Bach Flower Remedies alongside his orthodox treatment, which is why he approached a Bach practitioner for help.

Gordon arrived at the consultation in a state of near terror. His eyes were wide open and he was sweating heavily. He explained that his depression and anxiety left him unable to travel by himself. His father drove him to work as he was too frightened to take the bus - in fact his father had driven him to the consultation as well.

Gordon said that he kept his fears hidden from his co-workers, and pretended to be happy and cheerful so that they would not find out how he really felt. He was going out with a girl who was sympathetic to his plight, but he felt guilty because of the effect that his problems were having on their relationship.

The first treatment bottle mixed for Gordon contained Rock Rose for the terror of travelling and of having an accident; Aspen for a generalised, vague sense of fear and foreboding; Agrimony for the way he tried to hide his real feelings; and White Chestnut because his thoughts were out of control and his mind was never still.

The next consultation took place a month later. He used the lift to get up to the practitioner's rooms, and started off by saying that it was the first time in three years that he had actually ridden in a lift. Generally the fears were less pronounced, although they still surfaced from time to time.

After taking the remedies he now felt more aware of the source of his fears: it was the fear of being trapped that caused the anxiety.

He mentioned again feeling guilty over the effect that his fears had on his girlfriend, and also a general lack of confidence.

As the fear now had a definite name and cause he was given Mimulus at this time, and Pine was added for the guilt. The lack of confidence, which caused him to avoid challenges, indicated a need for Larch, and White Chestnut was again used to help calm his worrying thoughts.

Treatment with the remedies continued over the next few months. At each stage one or two new remedies were introduced to deal with newly-identified aspects of his mental state, and as the fear started to lessen so the importance of Larch grew. 'I think of all the remedies Larch was the one that helped me the most,' he told his practitioner. 'I have got back my natural courage to do things, and now I feel strong and fearless.'

EILEEN'S STORY

At 68, Eileen suffered from clinical depression. She had been taking a number of different anti-depressant drugs for more than three years, most recently Prozac. Despite this she remained very tearful. She suffered from loss of appetite, insomnia and anxiety, accompanied by digestive problems and a chronic stomach-ache.

At the first consultation Eileen appeared nervous and struggled to control her feelings when she talked about her problems. As the last of eleven children she had ended up taking care of her eldest sister's children and had missed out on school. She described herself as a shy and nervous little girl, and her childhood as full of panic, tears and stomach-aches. Since then she had married, moved to a new country, and had four children of her own, one of whom was autistic. This child lived in a residential home, and Eileen was eaten up with worry over what would happen to him after she was dead.

Knowing a little about her childhood made it easier in this instance to identify Mimulus as a probable type remedy for her - a selection that was backed up by her current nervousness and many incidental fears. Her extreme sense of hopelessness after having tried so many drugs with no improvement indicated Sweet Chestnut, and the various unresolved traumas in her past led the practitioner to include Star of Bethlehem as well. Finally, her worries over her son's welfare indicated the need for Red Chestnut.

The practitioner next saw Eileen when she dropped in about ten days later with the gift of a piece of cake as a thank you. At the next regular appointment she explained further what had happened to her. Following her third day on the remedies her appetite had started to come back - which accounted for the freshly-baked cake. Her stomach had not hurt her once, and all the pain had gone. On an emotional level she felt calmer and more alive, so that she was able to enjoy her grandchildren more.

No further remedies seemed necessary. There was no relapse, and with her doctor's co-operation Eileen was able to plan a reduction in her use of antidepressants.

KAREN'S STORY

Karen was referred to a Bach practitioner by a friend of hers who was a client of the same practitioner. During the consultation she was quietly spoken and reasonably calm, but as she spoke tears came to her eyes every so often, and she kept her head bowed.

She talked about her son, aged three, and the feelings that she felt towards him - feelings of anger and resentment, the latter based on the fact that she felt it was unfair that she could no longer enjoy her old lifestyle now that she had a child. She often lost her temper with him, then felt guilty and depressed at her own lack of control. Things were so bad that her son was starting to stutter, while she was more and more afraid to be left alone with him, for fear of what might happen.

It was important to reassure Karen that the negative thoughts that she was having about her son did not make a her a bad person - in fact she was taking a brave step by acknowledging the way she felt and seeking to do something about it. And it was important too to suggest that she seek out extra counselling from someone qualified in the area of child abuse and family relationships, as much for her own protection as for her son's.

Her fear of losing control of herself and doing harm to her son was a clear indicator for Cherry Plum. The resentment and bitterness about being trapped into the role of mother indicated the need for Willow, and the guilt and self-reproach that she felt over these unnatural feelings indicated Pine. In addition she was recommended to keep some Rescue Remedy to hand for herself and for her son, whenever the atmosphere between them became too tense. At the second consultation the relationship between Karen and her son had improved to the extent that they were enjoying each other's company more. Her violent, uncontrolled impulses had faded to a marked degree; and at the same time she had begun to see more clearly where these feelings were really coming from.

For the first time now Karen was able to talk about the sexual abuse she herself had received from her stepfather. She was full of hatred for this man, and at the same time, perhaps to compensate for the powerlessness of her early years, she tried to control other people. Holly and Vine were clearly indicated, and were added to the mix.

As the treatment progressed Cherry Plum was no longer needed, as she no longer feared doing violence to her son or being alone with him. However, Karen continued to take the other remedies for some time. They were no longer needed specifically for the relationship between her and her son. Rather, they were helping her to come to terms with her feelings about her stepfather - feelings which were being brought to light in a series of independent counselling sessions.

USING THE REMEDIES WITH OTHER THERAPIES

As some of these stories suggest, people often use the remedies as a complement to other approaches to health. In some instances other therapies support the use of the remedies, in others the remedies take a secondary and supporting role to the other approach. In either case the remedies focus on the emotional and spiritual state of the person, and do not interfere with other interventions, whether orthodox or alternative, spiritual or physical.

Complementary health professionals in many different disciplines frequently use the remedies in a similar way, as a helpful addition to their main therapy. For example, someone who is giving aromatherapy massages might choose to add one or more remedies to the massage oil. Even better, she might give her client a treatment bottle to take away with her. That way her client gets the continuing benefits of regular Bach Flower Remedy use in between actual sessions on the massage table.

More and more orthodox medical practitioners – particularly people who have daily hands-on contact with patients, such as midwifes, nurses and general practitioners - are also seeing the benefits of using the remedies alongside their drug- or technology-based approaches. Patients find comfort from having something to hand that they can take as often as they need, and the remedies help to treat the underlying causes of stress while the physical fall-out is eased using more direct intervention.

This kind of complementary use can be recommended in the vast majority of cases. The remedies themselves are non-toxic and will not react or interfere with other medicines. The only possible contra-indications are to do with the fact that they are preserved in alcohol - and even then the amount of alcohol taken can be reduced to near zero if the remedies are diluted before use.

We will learn how to dilute remedies before taking them later on, and will look more closely at the alcohol question later on. Before doing that, however, we will get a deeper insight into the remedies if we spend some time looking at a few basic concepts. What do the remedies actually do to us? And is it possible to go further, and explain how they go about doing it? We will try to answer these questions in the next chapter.

CHAPTER 3

HOW DO BACH FLOWER REMEDIES WORK?

SELF-HELP AND SELF-IMPROVEMENT

Ideally, a therapist who selects some remedies for you will want to teach you how to do the selecting for yourself. She will aim to encourage you to help yourself with the remedies – to encourage self-help. And if you buy a book on the remedies and start to use them without the assistance of a practitioner then you are taking the self-help route right from the start. But what exactly does self-help with Bach Flower Remedies really mean?

Many people read 'self-help' as 'self-improvement'. We are all familiar with the thousands of books on the market that promise a new you in twenty days, or that offer to advance your career, love-life, or spiritual or physical development to such an extent that you will not recognise yourself by the end of the last chapter. Self-help in many of these books means not being who you are. It means adopting a set of ideal characteristics that will make you someone else, it means copying someone else, or following someone else's blueprint. Self-help becomes self-annihilation: out with the old you and on with the new.

BEING YOURSELF

Bach Flower Remedies are different. Instead of a new you, the promise here is to introduce you to someone you might not have met for some time: the old you. Self-help in this conception means helping yourself to be yourself.

Or Bach believed that we are all here on earth to learn from who we are. Our time on the planet is an opportunity to discover our strengths and to work on our weaknesses. Doing this does not mean becoming someone else; instead, it means working to find out who we really are. It means finding the richness in being ourselves, rather than trying to be someone else.

THE HIGHER SELF AND THE PERSONALITY

Why should we want so much to be who we are?

The answer to this question lies in the belief that there is more to us than our everyday personalities. Dr Bach expressed this idea by breaking down the whole of people's emotional and spiritual beings into two complementary halves.

One aspect is the higher self - the spiritual aspect of ourselves, our soul, the divine spark. The higher self is immortal and perfect; its role is to allow the whole person to move towards perfection.

The higher self does not manifest directly in our lives. Instead it appears through the personality, the second of the two components that make up a whole person. The personality can be defined as our everyday mental life. It is here to help the higher self to achieve perfection for the whole. It does this by experiencing life and overcoming difficulties, gaining wisdom on the way. However, the personality has a limited autonomy of its own. Instead of completing its mission it can be led astray by outside influences, or itself fall into error, and begin to follow a path that diverges from that laid down by the higher self. The personality in this case has lost its way. It is no longer itself. It can be said to be out of balance with its own life's purpose.

THE CONCEPT OF UNITY

As well as being true to ourselves, which means being true to our higher selves, we also need to live in right relations with other people and with the universe as a whole. Viewed from the right angle we are all bound together: none of us is separate, but we all form part of a unified whole. It follows from this principle that if we are cruel towards another person then the wrong action will in the end come back against us. Anything that hurts another ends by hurting all.

This is easy to understand. It is perhaps less easy to see that one way of hurting other people is to try to control them. This is because each individual person has his or her own particular path to follow, and if we interfere and divert another into a path of our choosing then we are once again disrupting the overall harmony of the whole by causing other parts of that whole to misfire.

This is why when we seek to control or otherwise harm others we can be said to be out of balance with the unity of the universe.

IMBALANCE AND ITS RESULTS

There are therefore two faults that our personalities can commit. The first is to take a false path by not living the life that we are here to live. The second is to sin against the whole by hurting or impeding the life of another. Both lead to a state of imbalance.

When we are ourselves and are living at peace with others we are in balance. When we are not ourselves, or when we have given in to our weaknesses, or when we are at war with others, then we are out of balance.

Being out of balance means falling prey to sickness, because sickness and ill-health are the physical manifestations of this state. They can be seen as the higher self's attempt to rein in the personality and prevent it from going further off the rails. If the balance can only be brought back, then health will return, just as the sun shines in when the curtains are pulled back.

THE SNOWBALL EFFECT

That is the theory; now let's see how this process works in practice.

Imagine that you are working at a job you enjoy, making furniture. You do your work by hand and use the best-quality materials because that's what you enjoy. You work for yourself, don't answer to anyone, and you are making a comfortable living despite the fact that you would only expect to sell thirty or so pieces in a year. You have found your niche, and you are at peace with the world.

Your brother-in-law owns a medium-sized factory twenty miles away, which produces thousands of cheap, mass-produced sets of dining-room furniture. He too enjoys his work. For him satisfaction comes from the hustle and bustle of making deals and working with a team of machinists. He is also proud of the fact that his furniture really is value for money, and that it can be bought by people who could never afford the things you make.

One day your brother-in-law comes for a visit with the rest of his family. At dinner he notices the dining-room table, which you designed and made for yourself. Later, after mulling things over, he offers you a very large salary - more than double what you currently earn - to go and take personal charge of his design department.

You think it over. You don't want to do it, but you have always found it hard to say no to him, and it is a lot of money... Reluctantly you accept the offer.

At first you throw yourself into the new job, determined to make a success of it, and in the back of your mind is the thought that you will be able to keep making your own furniture in your spare time. But the hours at the factory are long and the journey to and from work takes up yet more time. By the time you get home the children are already in bed, and you barely have the energy to sit in front of the television. At weekends you try to make it up to the children. Your tools gather dust in the workroom.

Up to now you have got on well with your brother-in-law, in a distant kind of way. Now that you work for him, however, the relationship has subtly changed. He is very pleasant, but he expects you to do as you are told, and he can be fairly abrasive if he thinks you are not pulling your weight. And if you are honest with yourself you are not pulling your weight. Your first few designs are pretty bad, and look even worse when they have been knocked together out of the fibreboard and cheap pine that he uses for raw materials.

After a month or so you begin to suffer from headaches, and you find that you are taking out your frustrations on your family. You hate yourself for doing it, but you are permanently on a short fuse. You lose your temper before you have time to remember to keep it, and smack the children – something you never did in the past. You are tired all the time, and beginning to lose confidence in yourself as a father and as a designer.

Eventually your health breaks down into a series of colds and attacks of the 'flu. You feel sorry for yourself - it's all everyone else's fault; you begin to hate your brother-in-law for messing up your life, and you plan how you can take revenge...

This is a made-up case, but it shows how easy it is to be unbalanced by the things that happen to us in life. In the story, you were in balance when you were following your own path in life: making your furniture your way. Your brother-in-law was also in balance, doing work that he liked and making a positive contribution. The problem started when you allowed yourself to be deflected from your own path in life.

When your brother-in-law made the job offer you could have said 'no'; if you had taken the Centaury remedy this would have helped you to do so, and the potential problem would have been nipped in the bud and would never have occurred.

If, on the other hand, you only turn to the remedies when the problem is already there then you may have forgotten all about the fact that the real cause was your failure to resist someone else's wishes. Instead you will be suffering from a collection of apparently unrelated mental states: guilt for neglecting your children; guilt for not doing a good job; frustration; tiredness; even a lack of confidence in your ability to do your job at all. And after a time, as we have seen, these feelings may also be covered up - in our example by self-pity and hatred.

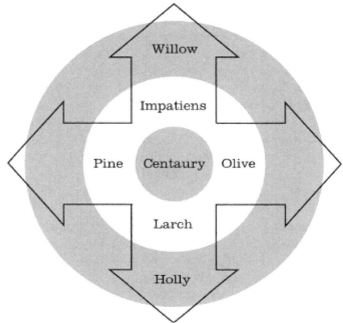

The Snowball effect: how emotional states build up in layers

This is what we mean by the snowball effect: the fact that untreated imbalances tend to lead to the build up of layers of negative emotions. Once the snowball effect has taken place you have lost sight of your path in life, and of the original problem, and there may seem to be so many emotional problems that need to be treated that you may be unsure where to begin.

PEELING THE ONION

How then is the snowball effect undone?

The ideal would be to take the one remedy that you need at the moment that the first threat to your balance comes about. If you had only taken Centaury when you needed to ...

But if like most of us you only begin to see the problem when the damage has been done, then a different process has to be followed, one usually referred to as 'peeling the onion'. This means removing layers of negative emotion one by one, so as to work back gradually to the core problem.

Peeling the onion: the remedies work from the outside in, until – the real root of the problem is revealed

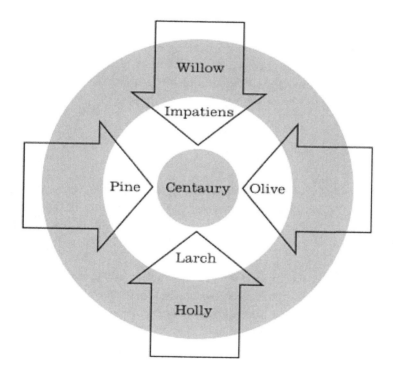

So in the above example you might take Holly and Willow first, in order to resolve your bitterness and remove the desire to take revenge against your innocent relative. Once this has been achieved you will see again what is underneath the bitterness: your guilt at treating your children badly, your frustration, your tiredness. You take the remedies for these states and, in time, the underlying cause - the Centaury state - will also be revealed. Finally you take the remedy for this and you can see again where your true interests lie, and take steps to put yourself back on your own path instead of following your brother-in-law's.

This can be a slow process where there are many layers of emotional baggage to work through, but it is a valuable one. Using Bach Flower Remedies is in the end a process of learning about yourself. Peeling the onion gives us the chance to learn from our mistakes, so that we are less likely to repeat them in the future. And it also means that we do not need to analyse ourselves into the ground right at the start. Instead we can take the remedies we need now, and let the remedies do the work of uncovering the hidden heart of our situation.

REGAINING BALANCE

As we have seen, the remedies work to peel the onion and so reveal the initial imbalance. They then help to restore balance so that we are once more ourselves and can resume our course in life.

This means that the action of the remedies is restorative, in that they work to bring us back to who we were when things began to go wrong. This in turn allows us to continue our personal path of growth and evolution.

However, we saw at the start of this chapter that people sometimes interpret the action of the remedies in a different way, and see them not as restorative but as aspirational- in other words, actually carrying out the growth and evolution for us, helping to turn us into something else. To see how false this idea is we only have to look at what happens when people take remedies. A shy, timid person taking the correct remedy will regain that natural quiet courage that will allow him to face up to things instead of running from them, but he will not turn into a flamboyant daredevil. Indeed, if a person were to taken some potion to change his nature in this way he would only be making himself even further out of balance in a different direction.

There is no short cut to personal development. Growth can only take place when we are back in balance and able to carry on living and learning from our lives. This is what evolution means: living and learning. And balance itself is not to be found at the extremes of our ups and downs. Instead it lies at the midpoint of the seesaw, where we are who we are.

VIBRATIONS AND ENERGY

The obvious question that arises is, how exactly do the remedies work? What is the mysterious force that restores balance to out-of-balance emotions?

There have been various theories put forward over the years. In Dr Bach's day people talked about 'vibrations' and described how the vibrations of a prepared remedy echoed the natural vibrations of positive emotions. Dr Bach himself talked about vibrations at different times, although unlike some of the theorists he did not pretend that he knew what a vibration really was - it was just a name given to a force.

More recently the talk is of 'energy' or, more often, 'subtle energy'. This is a form of energy that we have not yet succeeded in quantifying, and one which works on the spiritual and mental plane - sometimes referred to as the 'subtle body'. Dr Bach made a very clear statement about theorising at the end of his research. 'They who will obtain the greatest benefit from this God-sent gift,' he wrote, 'will be those who keep it pure as it is; free from science, free from theories, for everything in nature is simple.'

The message of this statement is clear: theories as to the way the remedies work do not help us to use them effectively. In fact all of the theories so far advanced have not helped anyone to use the remedies better. However much they try to incorporate fashionable scientific concepts like quantum mechanics and chaos theory they remain untestable and function purely as metaphors: you are at liberty to pick the one that seems most satisfying to you, but that does not mean that the metaphor you choose is truer than any other.

The remedies, for the moment at least, remain part of that wide range of phenomena that we can use every day but for which we have no understandable explanation. From consciousness to gravity to aspirin we have no idea why the basics of our universe function. If the action of the remedies appears strange and unaccountable, they are at least in good company.

LIKE BEAUTIFUL MUSIC

In fact the best metaphor for the action of the remedies ('best' in the sense of being the one that has the most explanatory power) is probably Dr Bach's own. He spoke of the remedies as being 'like beautiful music, or any gloriously uplifting thing which gives us inspiration.' Their action serves to 'open up our channels for reception of our spiritual self.'

This is a good analogy. If you listen to a piece of music that means a lot to you - whether it is by Bach, Beethoven, Bing Crosby, The Beatles or whoever - you are moved by it. Something that is in you already is stirred and called out by the music, so that you feel differently from the way you felt before. You are not changed from who you were, but a different side of your personality responds and is strengthened.

This is exactly what the remedies do. They do not put emotions into you that were not there before. Instead they encourage the positive emotions that are already in you, so that they become strong enough to overwhelm and drive out the negative emotions that were dragging you out of balance.

The music metaphor is in fact so good that it can explain other aspects of remedy use that may appear at first to be counter-intuitive.

For example, many people coming to the remedies for the first time are confused by the dosage instructions. They cannot see how taking two drops of pure remedy straight from a stock bottle can possibly be the same as putting the same two drops into 30mls of water and then taking only four drops of that extremely dilute mixture. If the remedies worked like orthodox drugs (the line marked 1 in the illustration), the stronger mix would have a stronger effect; and if they worked like homoeopathy (marked 2), then the more dilute dose would be stronger. Yet with the remedies both doses are the same. How can this be?

A melody is a melody: the effect of different strength doses

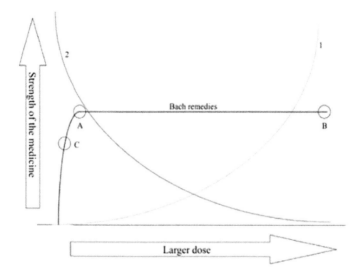

Again, the answer comes when we think of the remedies as music. A melody is a melody whether it comes from someone playing a flute three streets away, or from a symphony orchestra right in the room with you. If you can hear the melody you can hear the melody, and the volume is irrelevant.

In the same way, if you are getting the minimum dose of a remedy - four drops from a treatment bottle, marked A in the illustration - then we could say that the message the remedy is sending is just within earshot. You do not hear it any better if you take drops straight from the stock bottle, or even drink down a whole stock bottle (B) - it may be louder but it is still the same melody. And if you take less than the minimum dose - say two drops from the treatment bottle instead of four (C) - then you can no longer hear all the melody, and the remedies do not work as well.

The same analogy also helps us to understand what is happening when we mix remedies together. Selecting the remedies we need and mixing them together is like mixing the different melodies into a musical arrangement. If you have chosen the right ones the piece of music comes through very strongly and is easy to hear. If you put in a couple of remedies that you don't need then the sound of those remedies makes it harder to hear the notes produced by the others. And if you mix too many remedies together - more than the recommended six or seven - then you will have real trouble picking out the necessary notes at all.

A harmonious selection of remedies

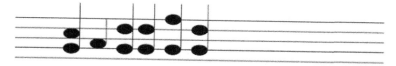

Too many remedies

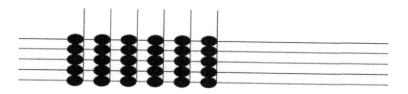

In Dr Bach's day someone suggested that he might combine all his remedies to produce a single elixir for everyone. He tried this, and found that mixed together like this the remedies did not work. In the same way, playing all the notes available all at the same time produces white noise, so that no music can be heard at all.

ARE BACH FLOWER REMEDIES PLACEBOS?

The remedies, like other forms of complementary medicine, are sometimes accused of being nothing but placebos. Sceptics say they only work because the person taking them thinks they will work. The same results would. be achieved if there were no flowers used at all.

There is a measure of truth in this, but only to the extent that all medicines and therapies, including the strongest of orthodox drugs, also have a placebo effect. In fact, a placebo effect is the power of positive thinking. If you think something is good for you then you will feel better. When you have a headache and take an aspirin part of the effect of the aspirin is to build up your confidence that the headache will go.

The strength of the placebo effect can be demonstrated by looking at its opposite - the nocebo effect. The nocebo effect is the power of negative thinking. It takes place when a drug that we know works is given to someone who believes either that the drug does not work, or that it is only a dummy drug. If you took an aspirin believing it to be nothing but a sugar pill, for example, then the nocebo effect would mean that the chances of your headache going would be reduced.

The nocebo effect probably explains why people who believe in witchcraft or black magic are at risk from sorcerers. Their belief in the power of spells is such that they really do fall ill and die if someone lays a curse on them. It can also explain why the remedies may not always help people who refuse to give them a fair trial. Sceptics who approach the remedies firmly convinced that they do not work are more likely than others to have their prejudices confirmed. In this they are no different from people who do not believe in the power of aspirin, or antibiotics, or radiotherapy...

There is of course more to orthodox medicine than belief, and again the same is true of the remedies. This is shown by the fact that they work on people who do not believe in them. Sceptics have been helped despite themselves, and people who have been given the remedies without their knowledge have also benefitted. (It may not be morally defensible to treat someone without consent, but it is not unknown between husband and wife ...)

Furthermore the remedies have been shown to be effective with animals and plants, and with very young babies, as we will see in chapter seven. It cannot easily be shown that animals and babies respond to suggestion, so the conclusion must be that they are potent in their own right, over and above the placebo effect that they share with all therapies.

CHAPTER 4

THE REMEDIES

Now that we know something about the background to this system of medicine, we can look in more detail at the individual remedies that go to make it up. There are 38 in all, plus the so-called '39th' remedy, with which we will start. ..

RESCUE REMEDY

The best-known remedy in the Bach Flower Remedies range is called Rescue Remedy. Rescue Remedy is not in fact a remedy at all, but instead a mix of five remedies, as follows:

• Star of Bethlehem - for shock
• Rock Rose - for terror
• Clematis - for faint, far-away, disconnected feelings
• Impatiens - for agitation
• Cherry Plum - for loss of self-control

Rescue Remedy is unique in Dr Bach's system. He taught his colleagues not to use ready-mixed formulas, but instead to look at the personality and emotional state of each individual and select a personal mix on that basis. Nevertheless he was well aware that there would be times when something would be needed at once - emergencies when there would not be time to select specific remedies. Rescue Remedy was put together with occasions like these in mind.

Dr Bach had occasion to use the Rescue Remedy himself and always carried a bottle in his pocket. Once, when he was living in Cromer, a lifeboat rescued a man who had been strapped to a mast for five hours during a storm. Many thought the sailor would die - he was in a delirium and stiff with cold. Bach moistened his lips with Rescue Remedy all the way up the beach, and by the time they reached the first house the sailor was able to sit up and talk to his rescuers.

As well as being useful in this kind of crisis, Rescue Remedy is also used to help overcome less dramatic situations. Pre-exam nerves can be calmed by it, for example, or you can take it when you receive bad news or when you feel upset and in a state after an argument.

LINDA'S STORY

'I went into labour after being induced with Pitocin, a drug which is known to make labour particularly intense and painful. After only a little progress I felt overwhelmed with the pain and felt I could not take any more. I was feeling very scared and asked for pain relief.

'My labour assistant, knowing I wanted to get by without pain relief, suggested I use Rescue Remedy. I took a dose and by the very next contraction I had calmed down, focused on the job, and taken control. The pain didn't go away but I was able to manage it so that it didn't overwhelm me anymore.

'I took three or four more doses over the next five hours and gave birth to my son completely without pain relief and completely in control of the birth. I am sure that the Rescue Remedy helped me get over my initial anxiety and so let me have a wonderful natural birth experience. I am recommending it to all my pregnant friends.'

GOING BEYOND RESCUE REMEDY

Because it is a remedy for emergency use Rescue Remedy is not really mixed with the intention that it be used long-term. If you find you need rescuing on a regular basis then it is a good idea to think about why this might be, and so start to identify the particular remedies that you need to solve the root of the problem. Rescue Remedy will help calm your exam nerves, but if your exam nerves are rooted in a chronic lack of confidence, or if you are nervous because you have once again failed to revise properly, then there are other remedies that would apply and which would do more long term good.

Rescue Remedy should not be a quick fix that you take to keep you functioning in your old out-of-balance way, but a gateway to those 38 individual remedies that can actually put your life back into balance.

THE SEVEN GROUPS

In his final publication of his work, The Twelve Healers and Other Remedies, Dr Bach sorted the 38 remedies into seven groups, as follows:

- remedies for fear
- for uncertainty
- for insufficient interest in present circumstances
- for loneliness
- for over-sensitivity to influences and ideas
- for despondency or despair
- for over-care for the welfare of others

You don't need to know which remedy is in which group, because in the end you simply pick the remedies you need regardless of the group they are in. Nevertheless, the groups can be useful to help understand some of the subtler differences between remedies, so we will come back to them again at the end of this chapter.

But for now it's time to look at the 38 remedies

REMEDIES FOR FEAR

Dr Bach grouped together five remedies under the heading 'Remedies for Fear':

• to treat fear of known things, things that you can name - Mimulus
• to treat terror - Rock Rose
• to treat fear of unknown things, things that you are not able to name - Aspen
• to treat the fear of losing your reason - Cherry Plum
• and to treat the fear that something will happen to a loved one - Red Chestnut

Mimulus

The plant used to make the Mimulus remedy is Mimulus guttatus, also commonly called the monkey flower. It grows in wet land, often at the edge of streams, and is remarkable for its large yellow flowers.

Mimulus is the remedy given to dispel everyday fears and anxieties, such as the fear of losing your job, or of speaking in public, or of the dark. In general, the Mimulus fear is any fear where you can name the thing that you are afraid of.

Mimulus is also associated with those types of people who tend to be nervous and shy, and who may blush easily or stammer. The remedy is taken to encourage the quiet reserves of strength and courage that lie underneath such everyday fears, so that anxieties can be faced and learnt from and overcome.

Rock Rose

The Helianthemum nummularium flower used to make Rock Rose is small and paper-thin, and coloured a translucent yellow. The plant itself grows close to the ground, often in stony or chalky soil.

As a remedy, Rock Rose is given to those who are suffering from a very great terror. The Rock Rose state is one of paralysis. Whatever is happening is so frightening that the person is incapable of dealing with it.

The aim in taking this remedy is to reawaken the will so that the terror can be faced and any necessary actions taken. Dr Bach used to refer to this as 'the remedy of emergency', so it is no surprise that it is one of the remedies he put into Rescue Remedy.

Aspen

Catkins from the Aspen tree - Populus tremula - are the essential ingredient of the Aspen remedy. The remedy itself is taken to counteract those vague, free-floating anxieties that seem to come for no reason. Sometimes the Aspen state can be one of real terror, but again no reason for the fear can be identified.

Instead it seems to consist of vague feelings, or superstitious dread with no real focus to it.

Contrast this state with the Mimulus fear, which always has a real, named cause.

The remedy works to strengthen your ability to trust life and trust yourself, so that you can come to see how faith can overcome any fear.

Cherry Plum

Cherry Plum comes from the spring blossoms of the tree Prunus cerasifera. The flowers are a beautiful sight, as white as snow and as numerous as snowflakes. They are all the more welcome for being among the first to appear just as winter is ending. The Cherry Plum remedy is taken to alleviate a very particular kind of fear, namely the fear of loss of reason and self-control.
The person in this state may fear that she is about to go crazy and injure herself or someone else.
A good example of this state is seen in toddlers who are having a temper tantrum. Their feelings overwhelm them, and underneath everything lies a great fear, caused by the intensity of their emotions and by their inability to control them.

The action of Cherry Plum is to give the person taking it the courage to confront his feelings and the causes of them. In this way the emotional crisis becomes an opportunity for learning and moving on.

Red Chestnut

Red Chestnut is another remedy for a very particular kind of fear, in this case the altruistic fear felt over the well-being and safety of someone else. Anxiety like this can become exaggerated and become a burden not only to the worrier, but to the person being worried about.

The remedy is made from the pink-red flowers of Aesculus carnea. Its action is to allow you to be concerned in a constructive way about the people you love, so that you can be a source of strength for them and so increase their self-confidence and faith in their own abilities.

There are six 'Uncertainty' remedies, as follows:

- for doubting your own decisions - Cerato
- for not being able to take decisions - Scleranthus
- for feeling discouraged - Gentian
- for pessimism and for giving up - Gorse
- for when you feel tired at the thought of the things you have to do - Hornbeam
- and for uncertainty about your true path in life - Wild Oat

Cerato

Cerato is an oddity among the 38 remedies as it is the only one that is made from a cultivated plant: Ceratostigma willmottiana. Originating from the Himalayas, in Britain it only grows in gardens like the one at the Bach Centre, where it has to be covered over each winter to protect it from the frost. The flowers appear in the summer and are an intense blue.

The remedy made from this plant is taken by people who lack faith in their own judgement. They make decisions but, having made them, immediately doubt whether they are doing the right thing. This leads them to ask other people for advice, which in turn results in their being led astray. Cerato acts to encourage your natural faith in your own intuition, so that you can act in the way that is right for you.

Scleranthus

The Scleranthus annuus is a tiny plant with green flowers, and can be very difficult to find because it blends in with the background. The remedy made from its flowers is taken by people who are having trouble selecting an option from among the alternatives in front of them. The decision in question could be about something important, such as whether to accept a new job or not, or about something relatively unimportant, such as whether to wear this jacket or that - but in all cases the

Scleranthus person dithers, first choosing one option and then the other.

Scleranthus encourages our innate decisiveness, so that we can cut through this form of uncertainty and make choices calmly and precisely.

Gentian

Gentiana amarella, the autumn Gentian, is the plant used to make this remedy. The flower is a deep blue-purple, and grows in clusters on upright stems.

Gentian is taken by people who have suffered a setback of some kind - an illness, for example, or failing an exam - and as a result feel discouraged and inclined to give up.

The effect of this remedy is to give encouragement so that you can quickly get over the setback and get on with your life.

Gorse

Gorse is made from the intense yellow flowers of Ulex europaeus, which is very common on exposed hillsides and heaths. The Gorse state can be thought of as being one step on from the Gentian state. If the Gentian person feels like giving up when life becomes difficult, then the Gorse person really does make up his mind to go no further. He decides that there is no way out, and adopts a pessimistic, hopeless attitude, even when other people suggest possible solutions to his plight.

Gorse is taken to give hope. It encourages your natural optimism to come to the fore, so overcoming the pessimism of the Gorse state.

Hornbeam

Hornbeam is made from the flowers of the tree Carpinus betulus. You take it when you feel weary simply at the thought of the work you have to do. For this reason Hornbeam is often referred to as the Monday morning remedy.

Hornbeam is also used when you find yourself putting off starting a job, and so is the remedy for procrastination. Hornbeam works to strengthen your determination to get started on the task in hand. Once this first step is taken the feeling of weariness melts away by itself, and the job can be completed without trouble.

Note that if you feel weary as a result of having done work then a different remedy is required - see the entry for Olive.

Wild Oat

The Wild Oat remedy is not in fact made from an oat at all, but from the wild grass Bromus ramosus. This only flowers for a very short time - a day or two at most - and as it is a sun method remedy we have to keep our fingers crossed that the weather will be kind at the right time. If it isn't then we just have to wait for next year.

You take Wild Oat when you are feeling dissatisfied and frustrated due to your inability to find your true path in life. Often people in the Wild Oat state will have tried many different paths in life, but nothing satisfies them. They know they want to do something worthwhile but are unable to say exactly what that something is.

The action of this remedy is to help us to listen more to our inner voice and take guidance from it. Deep inside we know what we are here to do, and Wild Oat can help us to identify that true path so that we can move ahead without delay.

REMEDIES FOR INSUFFICIENT INTEREST IN PRESENT CIRCUMSTANCES

Under this heading Dr Bach grouped seven different remedies, the indications for which are:

• to restore those who live more in dreams than in reality - Clematis;
• to restore those who live in the past - Honeysuckle
• to encourage vitality in those who are resigned to their lives - Wild Rose
• to restore strength to those exhausted in mind and body - Olive
• to quiet distracting, repetitive thoughts - White Chestnut
• to lift that type of gloom which descends from a blue sky - Mustard
• and to bring to mind the lessons of experience – Chestnut Bud

Clematis

The remedy Clematis is made from the cream-coloured flowers of the climber Clematis vitalba, which is more commonly known as Old Man's Beard.
This is the remedy used to help ground people who are not paying sufficient attention to the present because they are living in daydreams, either of an imaginary alternative reality, or of how things will be in some vague future.

True Clematis types may tend to fall asleep at odd moments during the day, and like to create magnificent plans in their heads that they never actually carry out in the real world. The effect of taking this remedy is that your inner drive and sense of purpose are anchored more to the present. Consequently, plans can be put into effect and more interest taken in the continuous present of life.

Honeysuckle

The plant used for this remedy is the wild pink honeysuckle, Lonicera caprifolium. The remedy itself can be thought of as the opposite of Clematis, for while the Clematis person is lost in daydreams of the future the Honeysuckle person is lost in remembrance of the past.

People in this state feel that their happiness lies all in the past. They are nostalgic, and miss out on chances to be happy today because of being wrapped up in yesterday. Sometimes they feel regret about something in the past, and this is what causes them to dwell on their memories of the way things used to be.

The Honeysuckle remedy, like Clematis, makes it easier for you to turn your thoughts and energies to the present so that you can begin to live today. You will not forget the past but will be able to learn from it and then move on.

Wild Rose

The dog rose Rosa canina is a familiar sight in many hedgerows around Britain, and this is the plant Dr Bach chose for the Wild Rose remedy.

Wild Rose is the remedy for apathy and resignation, for when we feel inclined to shrug our shoulders and accept whatever life throws at us without a struggle, instead of trying to make things better.

True Wild Rose types drift through life. They tend not to feel extremes of happiness or unhappiness, but just get on with whatever they have ended up doing. At times they can feel that life is passing them by, and it is then that the Wild Rose remedy is indicated. Its action is to awaken the sleeping sense of vitality and interest in life that lies under the surface of even the most disinterested of people.

Olive

Olive is one of two remedies that are prepared outside the United Kingdom - the other is Vine. It is made from the tiny white-green flowers of Olea europaea, which grows in many parts of Mediterranean Europe.

Olive is one of the most commonly used of the remedies. It helps restore spiritual and emotional energy when these have been exhausted by an effort of some kind. The effort concerned can be physical - such as exercising, hard work, recovering from illness - or mental, such as studying too hard.

White Chestnut

White Chestnut is another widely-used remedy. It is made from the white flowers of Aesculus hippocastanum, the horse chestnut tree.

This is the remedy to take if your mind is obsessed by a repetitive thought of any kind. The worrying thought could be a concern you have that is stopping you from thinking constructively, or preventing you from concentrating on something else; or it could be a scene from the recent or remote past that you are continually replaying in your head. In either case, the keys to identifying a White Chestnut state are: first, that the thought recurs despite your best efforts to stop it from doing so; second, that it is repetitive; and third, that it does not lead to a conclusion. The action of the White Chestnut remedy is to improve your mind's ability to remain calm and in control of its thoughts. This allows constructive thinking. If there is a problem that needs to be addressed then you are better able to find a coherent solution.

Mustard

The wild flower Sinapis arvensis is used in the Mustard remedy. Mustard is taken to treat the kind of down-in-the-dumps feeling that seems to come from nowhere, and for no reason. People suffering from this state may feel that life is full of good things for them, and that they should be happy - but they are not, and they cannot say why this should be.

The remedy works to reinforce our inner sense of joy and purposefulness, so that the negative clouds can disperse as quickly as they came.

Chestnut Bud

Chestnut Bud is made from the same tree as White Chestnut - namely the horse chestnut tree Aesculus hippocastanum. But while White Chestnut uses the flowers, Chestnut Bud is made early in the spring from the sticky buds, just at the point where they are opening up.

The time to take this remedy is when you feel that you are not learning from your own or other people's experiences and are repeating mistakes. (A friend is more likely to spot this tendency in you than you are yourself, since the Chestnut Bud state is one of unconsciousness and lack of insight.)

A typical Chestnut Bud state would be that of the person who ends a painful relationship with a violent partner, only to start a new relationship with another person with a similar history of violence. The lesson of life has not been learned, and it has to be repeated.

The action of Chestnut Bud is to help us to see ourselves and our actions more clearly so that we can grow and develop. And by watching and learning from others we may be able to avoid making a mistake in the first place.

REMEDIES FOR LONELINESS

The 'Loneliness' group is the smallest of the seven. Dr Bach listed just three remedies under this heading, as follows:

• to break down the walls that can build up around self-sufficient, independent people - Water Violet
• to bring patience to the impatient - Impatiens
• and to help self-centred, talkative people to understand the problems of others - Heather

Water Violet

The plant used to make this remedy is not in fact a violet at all - Hottonia palustris actually belongs to the primrose family - and 'violet' only refers to the colour of the five petals on the small, delicate flowers.

Water Violet is a type remedy for those people who like their own company and enjoy being self-sufficient and removed from the hustle and bustle of communal life. Other people may think them arrogant or snobbish, and this plus their natural reclusiveness can leave them isolated and lonely. The remedy frees up the great talents of people of this type, so that they can relate better to their fellow human beings and so put their wisdom at the service of others.

Impatiens

Only the pale mauve flowers of Impatiens glandulifera are used to make the Impatiens remedy - the darker flowers produced by some plants do not have the same properties.

As a mood remedy Impatiens is taken to relieve impatience and agitation in all its forms. The true Impatiens type is someone who keeps others away so that she can get on with her tasks faster. She is capable, intelligent and quick-witted, but in a negative state lacks the wisdom to see value in the more methodical talents of others.

The remedy acts to reinforce our hidden depths of patience and understanding, so that we do not need to go at top speed and can stop and appreciate life and the immense potential contribution of those slower than ourselves.

Heather

The Heather remedy is made from Calluna vulgaris, the mauve heather that grows across open moorland.

Heather is used to help people who have become wrapped up in their own affairs to the exclusion of everything else. They feel an overwhelming desire to tell other people every little detail of their lives, and for this they need to have an audience.

Or Bach referred to them as 'buttonholers' because they would literally catch hold of people to keep them listening.

Heather people fear loneliness. Unfortunately their incessant talking leads others to start to avoid them, so their behaviour brings about the very condition that they fear.
Taking this remedy helps to raise the mind above its own everyday concerns so that problems can be seen in context.

More interest can be taken in other people's lives, so that from being a great talker the Heather person can become a wise listener.

REMEDIES FOR OVER-SENSITIVITY TO INFLUENCES AND IDEAS

There are four 'Over-sensitivity' remedies, as follows:

- for pretending to be happy when underneath you are suffering - Agrimony
- for doing what other people want you to do and not what you should be doing - Centaury
- for protection against outside influences and the effects of change - Walnut
- and for feelings of suspicion, revenge and hatred – Holly

Agrimony

Agrimony - or Agrimonia eupatoria - is a long spiky plant covered in tiny yellow flowers. The Agrimony remedy is given to people who dislike disagreement and trouble, and so try to cover up any problems under a mask of good humour and cheerfulness. They appear happy even when they are suffering underneath, and will try to make a joke out of the most painful tragedy. Sometimes they will turn to drink or drugs to help keep the mask in place, and they may seek out company in order to forget themselves.

The Agrimony state appears brave, but it is really a way of not facing up to the darker sides of life. The remedy helps us to use humour to resolve situations, rather than using it to avoid them.

Centaury

Centaurium umbellatum is an upright plant with many small, star-shaped pink flowers. These are collected to make the Centaury remedy, which is taken by people who are having difficulty saying 'no' to others. Common examples of this would include the man who follows his father's choice of career rather than his own, and the woman who entirely gives up her own life to serve an ailing relative.

The action of the remedy is not to make us callous or domineering, but simply to allow us the freedom and strength to draw boundaries and mark out a place where we can live our own lives.Wecan remain willing helpers; but we will not be enslaved.

Walnut

The smaller female flowers of Juglans regia go to make up the Walnut remedy -, the larger male catkins are not used.
The remedy has two related uses. First, it is given to help people adjust to changes - people who are starting a new job or moving to a new house might use it to help them settle in, for example. It is equally useful during natural periods of transition such as teething and weaning and the menopause. In this aspect it is often called the link-breaker, because it helps ease the transition from one stage of life to a new one.

The second use is to give protection against outside influences that may lead us away from our path. For example, if you have decided to take a new job and live abroad, you may find that the negative opinions of your friends and relations are holding you back. This is the time to take Walnut.
The action of the remedy is to strengthen our self-belief and confidence. We are able to move ahead without being unduly affected by the thoughts and beliefs of others.

Holly

The tiny white flowers of Ilex aquifolium are much less well known than the famous red berries that develop from them, but they find a role in making up the Holly remedy.

This is given to help people who become suspicious of other people, and so develop negative feeling towards them, including hatred, envy and the desire to take revenge for actual or imagined wrongs. Holly is the remedy of love. It strengthens our understanding of other people and helps us to be open and generous even to those who really are acting wrongly towards us.

REMEDIES FOR DESPONDENCY OR DESPAIR

The 'Despondency or Despair' group is the largest of Dr Bach's seven groups. It contains the following eight remedies:

- to give us the confidence to try - Larch
- to help us be responsible for our actions without destroying ourselves with guilt – Pine
- to restore confidence when our responsibilities weigh heavily on us - Elm
- to give hope in even the darkest of nights - Sweet Chestnut
- to overcome shock and loss - Star of Bethlehem
- to lift us out of self-pity and towards generosity - Willow
- to give us the strength to go on and the wisdom to rest - Oak
- and to cleanse obsession and self-loathing - Crab Apple

Larch

The Larch remedy comes from the catkins of the tree *Larix decidua*, which is unusual in that it is the only conifer that sheds its leaves in autumn.

The remedy is taken to increase the confidence levels of people who are reluctant to try something because they are convinced they will fail. True Larch types feel that they are not as talented or capable as other people, and this can become an excuse for never trying to prove themselves.

The action of the remedy is to remove the fear of failure, so that the person can get more from life and not be worried by the eventual outcome.

Pine

The tree used to make the Pine remedy is the Scots Pine, Pinus sylvestris. It is a common sight in woodlands.

Pine is the remedy for guilt. When you are in a Pine state you tend to blame yourself for everything that goes wrong, and to go on blaming yourself even when everyone else has moved on. You may even assign blame to yourself when in fact someone else is at fault.

Pine works to replace the destructiveness of guilt with a more positive sense of responsibility and fairness. If something really is your fault you are better able to deal with it; and if it isn't then you will no longer carry the burden for other people.

Elm

Since Dutch elm disease arrived in the UK the common elm tree Ulmus procera is no longer as common as it once was. Fortunately a few colonies survive, and younger trees in many parts of the country can flower for many years before they eventually succumb to the disease.

As a remedy Elm is for the loss of confidence that comes when you have taken on too many responsibilities. The Elm state is one in which we doubt our ability to cope with all the demands being made on us. It can be usefully contrasted with the Larch state, which is also for lack of confidence. Where the Larch person is convinced of failure and so does not accept responsibility, the Elm person is usually capable and certain of success, and it is this that leads him to take on too much. The remedy works to restore our faith in our ability. The Elm state is usually a temporary one. Taking the remedy speeds it on its way all the faster.

Sweet Chestnut

This remedy is made from the long yellow catkins of Castanea sativa, the chestnut tree. It is given to people who have reached the end of the road and can no longer see any way out of their predicament. The Sweet Chestnut state is extreme, and once seen there is no doubt of it. It is the utter anguish of a bereaved parent, the complete despair of the man for whom not even suicide offers an escape.

There are no easy answers or quick fixes for someone in this state of mind. What the remedy can do, however, is to bring the tiniest ray of light into the darkness. This alone can be enough to bring comfort to the mental and emotional despair of the suffering person.

Star of Bethlehem

The white flower of the Ornithogalum umbellatum only opens up in sunlight. When night falls it closes up again. Star of Bethlehem is the remedy for shock and the after effects of shock. It helps to soothe the trauma associated with hearing bad news, or witnessing or being involved in accidents. By extension it is also used to help people who feel the pang of a great loss, such as the death of a loved one.

These indications explain why this remedy is a main ingredient in Rescue Remedy, and perhaps for this reason some people see

Star of Bethlehem itself as an emergency remedy for immediate use only. This is not correct, because Star of Bethlehem can also help us to come to terms with the effects of traumas that may have happened many years before, perhaps even in early childhood.

Star of Bethlehem helps our minds and hearts to get started again so that we can cope better with what has happened. It frees our will and lets us turn again towards hope and life.

Willow

There are many very similar varieties of willow tree around England and Wales, but the one chosen by Dr Bach for the Willow remedy was Salix vitellina. Known as the golden osier, it is so called because in winter the leafless twigs turn bright yellow.

The remedy is used to help people who are in a depressed state of mind in which they feel sorry for themselves and blame all their misfortunes on other people. They may feel resentment, feeling that life is not fair to them in particular and begrudge the success and happiness of others.

Willow helps to lift us out of this extremely negative state so that we can feel more generous about what other people do right, and more aware of the things that we ourselves are doing wrong. Left alone the negative Willow state tends to be selfperpetuating, as self-pity and resentment feed off each other; with the help of the remedy we can break the cycle and see things in a truer light.

Oak

The Oak remedy is made using the tiny scarlet-tipped female flowers of Quercus robur, the common oak; the much larger male flowers are not used.

Like the oak itself, which stands four-square in the countryside and supports more species than any other English tree, the Oak person is strong, slow and steady. She is a reliable type, able to take on immense responsibility and to work all hours without ever stopping or increasing her pace. Her immense strength is however the key to her downfall, because she does not know when she is exhausted and so struggles on long after she should have rested. This can lead to breakdown. Oak people never bend, but they can break.

The remedy works in two related ways. First, it helps to recharge our energies when we have exhausted ourselves with unceasing effort. Second, it helps us to measure our lives and efforts more sensibly, so that we can learn from what has happened and so give ourselves space to rest - and learn to rely on others from time to time.

Crab Apple

This remedy comes from the common hedgerow bush Malus pumila. The flowers are a delicate light pink inside, darker outside, and grow in clusters of half a dozen or so. Crab Apple is known as the cleansing remedy. We take it when we feel as if there is something unclean about our bodies or our appearance. For example, we might feel contaminated by an illness, or feel dirty and unattractive because of a skin complaint or a weight problem, and both situations would be ones where we might turn to Crab Apple.

By extension Crab Apple also helps to deal with contaminating thoughts and obsessive behaviours. Continual hand washing is the most obvious example, but in fact Crab Apple can be used to help any mental state where we are over concentrating on minor things and not paying attention to more important subjects. A candidate for this remedy would be the man who is obsessively pruning the roses around the door while the house falls down ...

People in a negative Crab Apple state can go to extremes of self-hatred, condemning themselves for what they are as well as how they look. In contrast, the remedy works to help us to accept ourselves and to see the essential cleanliness and beauty within. Living in a truer perspective we can concentrate more on things of lasting value and look less at appearance.

REMEDIES FOR OVER-CARE FOR THE WELFARE OF OTHERS

The last group contains five remedies, namely:
• when we want to be dose to our loved ones, and find it hard to let go - Chicory
• when we are filled with enthusiasm and want to convert other people to our way of life - Vervain
• when we force other people to do things our way - Vine
• when everyone else is stupid and wrong - Beech
• and when we strive for personal perfection, and to set an example - Rock Water

Chicory

The Chicory remedy is made from the beautiful blue-violet flowers of Chicorium intybus. This is the remedy to use when we feel that we want to cling on to the people we love, to keep them around us and focused on us. In order to keep ourselves in the centre of their attention we may offer unneeded help, or interfere, or act hurt and upset if we do not get all the attention we feel we deserve.

In a Chicory state we are full of love, but this love has turned inwards so that our own feelings are more important to us than the feelings of the people we want to help. The remedy allows our love to flow outwards, so that we can give without thought of reward, and feel happier because of this.

Vervain

Verbena officinalis is an upright plant with scattered clusters of tiny pale mauve flowers. The flowers go to make the Vervain remedy, which is used to treat states of over-enthusiasm. True Vervain types are perfectionists who throw themselves body and soul into whatever task or cause they are interested in. They are often full of energy, but their inability to switch off means that they can work themselves into the ground.

Vervain types like to persuade. They enjoy an argument, but when out of balance they begin to lose the ability to hear the other side, and their enthusiasm then shades into fanaticism. The remedy's action is to turn enthusiasm back into a positive attribute. It increases flexibility of mind, so that we can see other points of view without losing our own, and find value in stillness as well as in activity.

Vine

Like Olive the Vine remedy is made from a plant that grows wild in southern Europe and not in Britain. Vitis vinifera's fruit is the grape, and its tiny flowers are also green and grow in clusters. Vine is given to help people who sometimes use their talents and force of character to dominate others. Instead of trying to persuade, as a Vervain person would do, a negative Vine will not really care what other people think as long as they do what they are told.

The action of the remedy is to encourage the positive side of leadership, so that instead of being a tyrant the Vine person can be a guide, able to give freedom to others.

Beech

The beech tree Fagus sylvatica is a common sight in English woods, and we use its flowers - male and female - to prepare the Beech remedy.

The remedy is taken by people who find it difficult to sympathise with other people and their different lives. The Beech person is sure of the rightness of her life, and does not understand why anyone would want to live differently.

Beech people do not force others to change, but they do indulge in criticism, condemning what they do not understand instead of trying to see life through other people's eyes. The remedy does not affect the Beech person's sense of right and wrong or her high ideals. But it does help her to see the good within other people so that she can tolerate differences more easily. Back in balance, she is less tense and less irritable.

Rock Water

Rock Water is an oddity among the series of 38 flower remedies, because it is not actually made using a flower at all. Instead it is the water from an unspoilt healing spring - the one we use is in a remote part of Wales - which is prepared using the sun method.

The people who benefit from this remedy are those who turn their strictness and desire for control on themselves. They rule their own desires and set themselves rules and targets. They do not attempt to influence others directly, but indirectly they think that others might notice their example and be inspired to follow it.

When very out of balance the Rock Water person can become a martyr to his beliefs, taking a perverse pleasure in living a life devoid of pleasure. The joys of life are lost.

The remedy does not lower the Rock Water person's idealism, but it does bring it back into balance with his essential humanity. None of us can be gods here on earth. The remedy teaches the humility needed to be less than perfect.

USING THE GROUPS

As we said, you do not need to try to learn which remedy is in which group, but you can use the groups to help you understand some of the differences between remedies that at first sight might appear very similar.

Example one: Gorse and Sweet Chestnut

As an example we could look at the remedies Gorse and Sweet Chestnut. Key words given for Gorse often include 'hopelessness' and 'despair', but Sweet Chestnut is the remedy for people who have no way out of a situation and are feeling great anguish. They too have no hope and are in despair. So how do you go about deciding which remedy is appropriate?

One way is to look again at the groups that the remedies are in . Sweet Chestnut is in the group headed 'Despondency or Despair'. You might expect Gorse to be in the same category, but in fact it is grouped under the 'Uncertainty' heading.

How is Gorse a type of uncertainty? - The answer must be that people in a Gorse state lack a sense of conviction. They do not believe that they can get better, or do better, or find a way out of their predicament. Their problem is a lack of faith, and if they could regain their faith - their sense of inner certainty - then they would in fact be able to move on.

Sweet Chestnut, on the other hand, is for people who are genuinely in despair and without hope. They haven't decided to give up, as the Gorse person has, but have been forced into a corner where there is no way out of any kind. This is why this remedy, and not Gorse, appears in the 'Despondency or Despair' group.

Example two: Beech and Impatiens

Another example is Beech and Impatiens. Both remedies are given to irritable people, but again the groups they are in clearly signal the difference between them.

Beech is listed under 'Over-care for the Welfare of Others'. Beech people are concerned that other people are not doing things the right way, which in effect means their way. Because they are concerned they point out to people where they are going wrong. They criticise and condemn, but they show their care for others by taking the time to do this.

Impatiens on the other hand is a 'loneliness' remedy. Impatiens people do not care what other people do as long as it does not cause a delay. Instead of criticising a mistake they are more likely to take the job over and do it themselves so as to have it done quicker. They will not take the time to criticise, because they do not care how badly other people perform as long as it does not hold them up.

THE ORIGINS OF RESCUE CREAM

Rescue Cream is a homoeopathically-prepared cream that contains Rescue Remedy and Crab Apple. You use it on bruises, cuts, and skin problems of various kinds, as a quick and convenient way of applying the remedies externally.

At first sight the cream looks like a violation of the principle that the Bach Flower Remedies treat emotional states and not physical conditions. This is not in fact the case, but in order to understand the situation better it is helpful to go back to the origins of the cream.

When Dr Bach was working with the remedies he often used to apply them externally in addition to giving them as drops in the normal way. If someone suffering from eczema came to him he would look at the emotional state and select remedies on that basis. Vervain for over-enthusiasm, for example, perhaps combined with Olive for tiredness and Gentian for discouragement. He would prescribe these drops in the normal way and in addition he would instruct the person to use the same remedies in a cold compress to be applied externally to the affected area.

This is still done today, although in most cases the remedies are enough when taken internally, and for this reason most people use this method alone.

When people have an accident of some kind the first remedy to reach for is Rescue Remedy, and again it can be helpful, in addition to swallowing the drops, to dilute them and put them on the affected area. Just as Rescue Remedy is the most-used of the remedies, so it is the one that is most often used externally.

Rescue Cream was put together by Nora Weeks as a way of making it easier to apply the remedy to the skin. She added Crab Apple to the formulation because this is specifically the remedy that is given to people who feel that there is something wrong with their appearance; Nora felt that it would therefore be a useful addition to a cream precisely meant to be applied to bruises, rashes and so on.

Therefore, the cream is not specifically for the physical symptom, but is simply a way of addressing the physical aspect of what is still essentially an emotional trauma. Having said this, wonderful results have been achieved that show just how closely emotional and physical health are linked.

HESTA'S STORY

'Due to an accident my foot has had an open wound for 18 years. I've had several skin grafts, five in total, but none totally successful.

'I bought and tried Rescue Cream and in a matter of days I saw a difference. Now, seven weeks on, my foot is healed - no more bleeding or worry in case of infection. It's unbelievable to me.'

CHAPTER 5

HOW DO I SELECT THE RIGHT REMEDIES

THREE PRINCIPLES

There are three important principles to remember when selecting remedies for yourself. The first is that you are not selecting remedies for a disease. If you have a particular illness then for the purpose of using Bach Flower Remedies you need to ignore it.

This can be difficult to do. When people ask 'how are you?' it is natural to talk about aches and pains. But the remedies are selected purely for emotional states and personality problems. This means that when you have a cold you might end up taking the same remedies as when you have a cough. It also means that the next time you have a cold you might need different remedies. It doesn't matter: ignore the physical problem and look only at the way you feel about yourself and your life. (You can use other forms of medicine to help your immediate physical symptoms; and of course you should consult a doctor if you are worried about your physical state of health.)

The second basic principle is that you should select remedies for the way you feel now. The fact that you were depressed last Tuesday is irrelevant if you do not still feel depressed today. And the third principle is that you should treat what you see.

You do not need to subject yourself to lengthy psychoanalysis in order to select remedies. Instead you can stay on the surface and select remedies for what is obviously there. If there are deeper problems that need to be resolved these will become apparent as the remedies resolve the surface problems. (Remember the onion peeling process?)

So the three principles are these:

• ignore physical symptoms
• look at how you feel today
• treat what you see

MOOD REMEDIES

Impatience, intolerance, lack of will, apathy, self-pity, a sense of loss, discouragement, guilt, fear ... all of us at different times of our lives will experience all 38 of the remedy moods. When we do so we simply pick the remedy that we need at that moment. By doing this we are using the 38 remedies as mood remedies, and because they can all be used in this way we can say that all of the remedies are mood remedies.

Sometimes, when a short-lived mood is involved, it may be enough to select and take a single remedy. You quickly get over the negative mood and you do not have to take the remedy again.

But moods can be longer-lasting, in which case they may form part of a selection of remedies designed to resolve a particular negative mind-set that we are experiencing. In this case they are often mixed with a type remedy.

TYPE REMEDIES

So what is a type remedy? Put simply, a type remedy is one that describes your actual character. It says how you usually react rather than simply saying how you happen to be reacting at the moment.

We have seen that all the 38 remedies can be mood remedies. When it comes to type remedies, however, the situation is different. Star of Bethlehem is for shock, for example, Olive for tiredness, and Sweet Chestnut for anguish: these are clearly not descriptions of types of people.

So not all the 38 remedies are type remedies. Examples of the ones that definitely are would include:

• Impatiens - a remedy for the type of person who lives life in a rush, loses patience easily, and reacts to pressure by going faster

• Beech - a remedy for the type of person who often criticises others, and does not see value in other ways of life

• Centaury - a remedy for the type of person who finds it hard to refuse to help other people, who is easily taken advantage of and cannot say no

• Vine - a remedy for the type of person who will force other people to do things his way, and will not take no for an answer

These are just examples. If you read back through the remedy indications in Chapter 4 you will see many other remedies that seem to describe types of people and permanent characteristics, as much as they can describe temporary moods.

In practice there is no definite, fixed list of type remedies. This is because some such as Willow and Honeysuckle inhabit a kind of grey area. They may at first appear to be type remedies, but almost invariably the emotional states they describe turn out to be outer layers of the onion, with the real type hidden underneath.

FINDING YOUR TYPE REMEDY

In a sense, finding your type remedy is unimportant. As long as you follow the basic principle of treating what you see then you will always select your type remedy when you need to do so. Nevertheless, most people using the remedies like to take some time to work out what their type remedy is, because the type remedy tells you something about who you are and about the main weaknesses that you need to work on. Here then are a few tips to help you think about what your type remedy might be:

• Imagine yourself in a potentially stressful situation, such as working to a very tight deadline or taking 20 young children to the seaside for the day. How do you go about trying to organise things? How good are you at it? And what do you do when things go wrong?

• Think about your faults - or ask a friend to list them for you. What is the one thing that you need to work on most?

• Think about the qualities that you admire in other people. Are they qualities that you share or qualities that you aspire to?

• Imagine you have to accompany your partner to a formal dinner where you will not know anyone. How do you feel about the prospect? How will you behave on the night?

Answering these kinds of questions and comparing your answers with the indications for the remedies can help you to get on the track of your type remedy. Nevertheless, don't be too worried if you cannot work out your type straight away.

Remembering the onion again, there is no reason to believe that you need to be able to see its centre when you are only peeling away the first layer. As you take remedies for successive layers your true type remedy will become clear to you.

CAN YOUR TYPE CHANGE?

The type remedy describes your fundamental character, and as such your type remedy will not change over your lifetime. That said, you may well feel that it is changing. This is because at every layer of the onion there is the potential to be acting as if you were a different type.

Thinking back to the example of the furniture maker, his type remedy when he is out of balance and losing patience with his children may appear to be Impatiens. If he stays in this state for a long time he may forget that he was ever any different. As he begins to peel the onion, though, the Impatiens state will fade eventually - in fact it was simply a long-standing mood. His real type may be something completely different; Centaury, perhaps, or Walnut or Water Violet.

Most of the time people can eventually be pinned down to one clear type remedy. In some cases, however, this does not seem to work, and a combination of type remedies seem to be equally important. People are mixes of Mimulus and Impatiens, for example, or Vine and Vervain. In any case, the basic rule still applies: treat what you see, and the type (or types) will eventually come into focus.

SELECTING A PERSONAL MIX

How then does one go about selecting the remedies that are needed?

At first it can seem difficult. It is a commonplace among practitioners using Bach Flower Remedies that at first many people think that they need to take all 38, and find it very hard to cut down the selection. The way to do this is to apply the three principles that we saw earlier. To remind you, these were:

- ignore physical symptoms
- look at how you feel today
- treat what you see

So, once you have looked through the list of remedies and made a note of the twenty or so that seem to apply, the first thing to do is to forget about physical symptoms. You don't need to take Crab Apple (the cleansing remedy) every time you catch a cold - you only need it if the cold makes you feel contaminated and 'dirty'.

You then discard all the remedies that are for the way you felt last week. Only leave the ones that relate to the way you feel now.

Then you take out any that are based on guesswork - this is what we mean by 'treating what you see.' So if you think that there might be some shock in your background that explains your current depression, but you can't actually think what the shock might have been, then you don't need to include Star of Bethlehem. If the shock is really there and really relevant then it will appear more clearly once the initial mix of remedies has been taken.

Ideally you should take no more than six or seven remedies at a time. What do you do if you have applied these principles and still seem to have too many remedies in your list? The answer is to rank the remedies you have chosen in order of importance. So, for example, you might have chosen Vine because you recognise yourself in that description and think it is probably your type remedy - you have certainly been laying down the law at home for the past few days, and you can see that this is not the best way to go about things. And you may have chosen Gentian because you felt a bit down in the mouth this morning when you burnt the toast. It's fairly obvious that although both remedies do relate to today, Vine is more important than Gentian, so you can discard the Gentian.

Applying the same system of ranking to all of the remedies on your list you should easily be able to isolate those that are most important to you at this moment.

SHOULD I ALWAYS INCLUDE MY TYPE REMEDY?

Because your type remedy describes who you are and how you tend to react when things go wrong, most people usually end up including the type remedy in their mix of remedies. Does this mean that it is a good idea to always include your type remedy?

The short answer is 'no'. The same criterion applies as when selecting any other remedy: you only need to include your type remedy if it is apparent that you need it, and that you need it now. There would be no point taking your type remedy if you simply felt tired at the end of a long day and needed something to restore your energy; Olive alone would be indicated.

Even when mixing a treatment bottle there will be times when your type remedy is not involved in the way you feel. If it isn't needed, there is no need to take it.

WHAT IF I NEED A REMEDY THAT ISN'T IN THE SYSTEM?

Dr Bach said before he died that his system was complete, which means that it contains a remedy for every possible negative mental state that a human being can feel. How can this be true? Surely there are more than 38 negative mental states? And what do you do if you feel something that isn't covered by one of the 38 remedies?

Perhaps the best way to explore these questions is to draw an analogy with colour. There is an infinite number of visible shades of colour in the world. The computer I am writing on at the moment can only display 16 million of them, our eyes can distinguish many millions more. Yet all of them are made out of a mix of just three primary colours: red, blue and yellow.

In the same way there is an infinite number of different shades of emotion that human beings can feel. Yet all of them can be made out of a combination of just 38 basic states, and for every one of these basic states there is a remedy in Dr Bach's system.

If you sit down and do the mathematics (based on 39 remedies - 38 plus Rescue Remedy - and an absolute maximum of nine remedies in a mix) you will arrive at a little under 293 million available combinations.

In addition, two different people who need the same set of remedies will need them for different reasons. For example, George and his wife Jemima both need to take Impatiens and Mimulus, but their reasons for taking those remedies are very different. George is an Impatiens type who has said yes to making a speech without thinking it through. He has not had time to prepare, and now he is anxious about what will happen.

Jemima might be a Mimulus type who is dreading coming to the conference to hear the speech because it will mean having to meet lots of strangers afterwards. She needs Impatiens only because her fear is making her irritable about George's delay in writing the speech.

As this example shows, an apparently identical mix of remedies can actually cover many different mentalities. This is why we can claim that the 38 remedies, when used in combination, cover all possible mental states. And there is in fact empirical evidence for this claim: the Bach Centre has been recommending remedies to people since the 1930s, and has never yet had to send someone away because there is no remedy for their condition.

On a practical level, then, how do you cope when there does not seem to be a remedy for the particular problem that you have?

The answer is to break down the emotion to find out what it really means. For example, you may be suffering from stress. There is no remedy for stress per se, so you need to find out what stress means to you and why it is there. Are you stressed because you are trying to do everything too fast (Impatiens), or because you feel unfulfilled and can't find anything worthwhile to do (Wild Oat)? Are you putting yourself under stress because of your sheer enthusiasm (Vervain), or are you stressed because you have allowed someone else to control your life (Centaury)?

Similarly, there is no one remedy for anger. So if you are feeling angry you need to start by identifying the cause – intolerant Beech, spiteful Holly, indignant Vervain or resentful Willow - before you can select the right remedy.

The same thing applies to any feeling you have that does not seem to be covered. With a little thought you can quickly identify the remedies you need.

CHAPTER 6

HOW DO I TAKE THEM?

FOR PASSING MOODS

It's Monday. You come home after a day's work feeling tired, and you snap at the children for making too much noise. You need to take some Olive and Beech to help you out of this mood so that you can enjoy your evening. Here's how to do it:

1 Put some water in a glass

2 Add two drops of Beech and two drops of Olive to the water 3 Sip from the glass until you feel better

If you were including Rescue Remedy in the glass you would add four drops of that remedy, in addition to the two drops of each single remedy.

You can put the drops into any other drink instead of water if you prefer - the remedies are not like classical homoeopathic medicines, which cannot be taken alongside coffee and tea.

On the whole the remedies work quickly in this sort of situation, and taking the remedies like this is certainly the easiest way to prevent negative emotions from hanging around too long.

MIXING A TREATMENT BOTTLE

What if you are dealing with a more long-term problem and need to take the same mix of remedies for several days or weeks?

The answer is that you can if you want use the same system. Just -mix the remedies in a glass of water and sip from it throughout the day, and at least four times during the day. Then you make up a fresh glass each morning. But there is another method you can use that is more economical and in the long run easier, and that is to make up a treatment bottle.

A treatment bottle is simply a small medicine bottle containing water and the remedies that you want to take. Here is how to mix one up:

1 Get an empty 30ml (one ounce) dropper bottle. A dropper bottle is a bottle with a pipette built into the lid - you should be able to get one the same place that you buy remedies. If you can't get a 30ml bottle any smaller size will do

2 Put two drops of each selected remedy into the bottle (and four drops of Rescue Remedy if you are including that in the bottle)

3 Top up with mineral water - use the non-gassy kind so that it will not spill over the top

From this mixed treatment bottle you need to take four drops at least four times a day - ideally spacing the doses out during the day, with the first one on waking and last before you go to bed. You can take the four drop dose more often if you need to.

To take the remedies, drop the drops straight onto your tongue. Some people prefer to drop them under the tongue, which is fine as well. You can also put them into a teaspoon of water, or even take them in tea or coffee or fruit juice - as long as you get the four drop dose into you.

Treatment bottles are useful because they are easy to carry around with you, and they mean you can take a dose of your personal mix whenever you want to, quickly and easily. They will also save you a great deal of money because you are using much less remedy than you would be if you were making up remedies in a glass each day.

If you take the drops regularly the remedies in a 30 ml treatment bottle will last up to three weeks. To keep the water fresh for that long you can either keep the bottle in the fridge or add a teaspoon of brandy or any similar strength spirit to the water when you are mixing it up. Mineral water keeps best - if you use tap water it may go off, even if it is boiled. Distilled water should not be used as it is biologically dead.

If you get a couple of days into your treatment bottle and realise that there is another remedy that you need then simply add it to the mix - assuming this does not mean that you are taking more than seven or so remedies at a time. (For the purpose of counting the number of remedies, Rescue Remedy counts as a single remedy only.)

CAN I RE-USE A TREATMENT BOTTLE?

Even if you add brandy to your treatment bottle and keep it in the fridge, sooner or later the water will go off. This is because every time you open the bottle you are giving bacteria a chance to get into the liquid, and if you touch the dropper with your tongue then the water is certain to contain bacteria.

You can re-use treatment bottles, but because of the risk of contamination it is a good idea to sterilise them as far as possible before refilling them. To do this, first remove all the plastic and rubber parts. Then place the glass parts (the dropper and the bottle itself) into a saucepan of water. Heat the saucepan, and allow it to boil for between fifteen and twenty minutes. Remove the glassware and allow it to dry naturally. For a sparkling finish place it upside down in a warm oven. The plastic top and rubber teat can be washed in hot water. It is best not to boil them unless absolutely necessary as they will perish over time.

An alternative to boiling is to use one of the systems designed for sterilising babies' bottles. A steam steriliser is the best solution. Sterilising tablets are less good because they leave a residue in the bottles and can make the treatment bottles taste vaguely chemical.

IN AN EMERGENCY

In an emergency there is no time to make up treatment bottles, and there may not even be time to find a glass of water. In this case you can take drops straight from the stock bottle (the bottle you bought in the shop). The dosage is two drops on the tongue (or four of Rescue Remedy), repeated as necessary. What if someone has fainted and is unable to swallow? In this situation you can apply the remedies to pulse points or use them to moisten the lips or gums. This is not as good as taking them internally, but the effects of the remedies will still be felt.

OTHER USES

The remedies are designed to be taken internally, and the best results are always achieved using that method. Sometimes people like to use the remedies in other ways as well, though, usually as a back-up to taking them orally. The commonest techniques include using the remedies:

- in compresses
- as a lotion
- in the bath
- in sprays

To make up a compress, dilute two drops of each selected remedy (four of Rescue Remedy) into a small bowl of water. Use ice-cold water for swollen areas (you can add ice cubes as well if you want), or warm water for stiffened muscles and so on. Take a clean cloth, wet it in the medicated water and apply to the affected area.

For a lotion of remedies, just make up a glass of water with the remedies as you would do if you were going to take them by mouth. Then bathe the affected area in the water, or dab it on using a clean cotton-wool ball. This kind of use can be built into a regular cleansing routine if you are troubled with spots or other similar skin problems.

Some people have found that adding remedies to the bath can have a beneficial and relaxing effect. There is no exact dosage for this. Just put in three or four drops of each individual remedy and double that amount of Rescue.

Finally, you could add remedies to a water mister (the kind used to spray plants) and use this to freshen the room. A couple of drops of single remedies and four drops of Rescue Remedy should be sufficient.

All of these methods have been found to be useful, but it should be stressed once again that they are very much secondary to taking the remedies you need internally. That remains the quickest, simplest and most effective way of using them.

HOW FAST DO THE REMEDIES WORK?

Asking how fast the remedies work is a bit like asking how long it will take to climb a mountain. The answer is it depends on the size of the mountain, and it depends how quickly you are able to climb. Nevertheless there are some general rules that can be a guide.

First of all, and as you might expect, the remedies tend to work faster on moods than they do on more deep-rooted problems. This is why there are more dramatic stories told about Rescue Remedy than about any other remedy. People use it for acute crises which have thrown them off course. It can quickly correct this immediate imbalance and get you back to where you were.

Despite the occasional story of sudden cures and immediate relief, in general more deep-seated imbalances - the kind for which you would normally want to make up a treatment bottle - take longer to resolve. This is because they have taken root and become as if part of your personality. The more deep-rooted they are the longer the remedies will take to have an effect - but you would normally expect there to be some improvement after three weeks. If there is no improvement look again at the selection of remedies you are taking to see if it is as appropriate as you thought it was. Three weeks is about the time that a treatment bottle will last, so this is in any case a natural time to review your selection.

Often improvements are barely noticed, as imbalance tends to be more visible than balance. After all, if you have a headache you can think of nothing else, but when the headache goes you just get on with your life - you don't notice being well in the same way as you notice being ill. What this means is that you may not immediately see evidence of improvement unless you go looking for it.

You may only realise how far you have come when you think back to how things were when you started taking the remedies. Some people say that other people notice a change before they do. Comments like 'you're looking well' or 'you seem cheerful today' can be the first clue you have that the depression and stress that you were suffering have melted away.

ALLERGIES AND REACTIONS

People suffering from allergies sometimes ask if they can take the remedies. For example, someone allergic to aspirin might wonder if the Willow remedy is safe, as aspirin comes from willow trees; others might worry about taking Walnut if they are allergic to nuts.

If you look back at the first chapter of this book, you will remember that each remedy is indeed made using the plant named on the bottle, but that once the plant has energised the water the plant material itself is removed. In fact chemical analysis of the remedies shows that there is no actual plant-derived material in the bottle at all, and this is why people with allergies to the plants do not need to worry about using the remedies.

The only exception to this relates to the fact that the remedies are bottled and preserved in alcohol- but we will deal with that in more depth at the end of this chapter.

If the remedies do not cause allergies, what about reactions in other words negative or harmful effects? Again, the short answer is that the remedies do not cause reactions. They cannot, because they do not put into you anything that is not there already. Instead they simply enhance the positive side of your mental and emotional activity. They are wholly positive in their effect.

There is a longer answer, though, and this helps to explain where the idea of reactions to the remedies comes from.

As we saw in chapter 3, dealing with deep-rooted problems may involve working back through several layers of negative states before you can start work on resolving the fundamental imbalance. This explains why people sometimes complain that the remedies have caused not a state of balance, but a different state of imbalance. For example, someone who is taking Scleranthus for her indecisiveness may begin to feel critical of the people around her, and blame this on the remedy. What is happening, however, is that the layer of indecisiveness is being cleansed with the remedy, and the hidden feelings of intolerance, which may have been pushed away and hidden for many years, are now more clearly revealed.

The answer to developments like this is always to select remedies to deal with the revealed negative states. In this case Beech could be given either as well as, or instead of, Scleranthus.

A rather similar situation can arise when someone takes remedies and finds that the negative emotions seem to get stronger rather than weaker. This is simply because the remedy helps you to get your feelings into your conscious mind. Taking the remedies makes you more aware of how you feel, so that it can feel as if things are worse simply because you are more aware of them. The answer again is to persevere. As we have said, the remedies are only and always positive in their effect, and increased consciousness of a problem is the first step to resolving it.

Finally, and in extremely rare cases, people find that they have what appears to be a physical reaction to the remedies. When this happens it takes the form of minor rashes or rises in body temperature. In all cases the symptoms are mild and do not last long, and they are the physical signs of an emotional cleansing process taking place. If you are experiencing more pronounced symptoms, or if your symptoms go on longer than a day or so, then this has nothing to do with the remedies and you should consult your qualified medical practitioner.

Don't let all this talk of reactions put you off using the remedies. They are the safest and most gentle form of medicine around - so much so that they can be given (suitably diluted) even to newborn babies. You can use them without fear.

WHEN CAN I STOP TAKING THE REMEDIES?

The answer to the question 'when can I stop taking the remedies?' is quite straightforward. You can stop taking the remedies when you no longer feel that you need them. They are not habit-forming and you will not become dependent on them, so you do not have to wean yourself off. In fact many people find that when they no longer need their remedies they simply forget to take them.

Sometimes people continue to take their drops because they are concerned that if they stop the negative feelings will come back. This is not something to worry about. The remedies work to strengthen our positive emotions, and once they are strengthened they remain strong. It is a bit like mending a broken fence: you don't have to keep hammering once the fence is strong because it can stand by itself. If in a week's time a hurricane should come and blow the fence down, then that is the time to start mending it again. In other words, if something happens to throw you back out of balance then you can go back to the remedies then. They are always there to help.

In truth sensible use of the remedies need never stop. Once you have resolved any treatment bottle-scale problems that you have, then you can still use the system as mood remedies to keep you in balance whatever life throws at you. This was Dr

Bach's vision of how the remedies would be used: 'I want to make it as simple as this - I am hungry, I will go and pull a lettuce from the garden for my tea; I am frightened and ill, I will take a dose of Mimulus.'

A NOTE ON ALCOHOL

As we saw when we looked at the methods used to prepare Bach Flower Remedies, brandy is used as a preservative and as a liquid carrying medium for the energised water. We saw that every 10 ml stock bottle of remedy actually contains just two-thirds of a drop of mother tincture, while the rest is 27% proof brandy.

This fact can be a worry to parents who want to give remedies to their children but are concerned about the alcohol content. And it causes a particular problem for people who have decided not to drink alcohol, either for health or for religious reasons.

The first thing to stress is that if you dilute the remedies into a treatment bottle before taking them then the actual amount of alcohol involved is reduced almost to the point of not being there at all. Remember that a treatment bottle is 30mls of water plus two drops of each selected remedy, and that a dose from this bottle is only four drops.

This should be enough to reassure parents that diluted in this way even a small baby is not going to be affected by the amount of alcohol in a treatment bottle dose; but it will not help adults with religious or health objections to alcohol.

Some religions that ban the use of alcohol can make special dispensations for medical use. If you feel this might apply you need to approach your spiritual advisor for guidance on this point. Orthodox Jews have a particular problem in that the remedies are not kosher products, and again advice on this question should be sought from a rabbi. Even if taking the drops internally is not possible, the rules might allow you to benefit from the remedies by using them externally. Apply them to the temples, or wrists, or other pulse points.

Using the remedies externally can be an option for recovering alcoholics as well. Another is to put the treatment bottle drops into a very hot drink, which will evaporate almost all of the remaining alcohol. But when discussing the use of the remedies with people who do not want to drink, special mention needs to be made of a group of drugs that are sometimes given to recovering alcoholics to help them stop drinking. The most common of these is marketed as Antabuse, and like all the others it reacts to the presence of alcohol and causes the person who has taken it to feel extremely ill. Some reports have stated that even the use of alcohol-based aftershaves have caused reactions in susceptible people who have taken Antabuse. This makes even the external use of the remedies problematic, and again the best advice is to ask the person who prescribed the Antabuse in the first place.

Some people who have stopped drinking are reassured about using the remedies when they find out how dilute a treatment bottle dose is. But others who have sworn never to drink again may feel that even this trace amount of alcohol would represent a violation of the promise made, and the psychological impact of such a violation could be out of all proportion to the amount of actual alcohol involved. Certainly this is the position adopted by Alcoholics Anonymous, and it is one that should be respected.

In all cases where the alcohol content of the remedies is a problem the final decision must be left in the hands of the person who is considering taking the remedies. All of us who use them to help others have a duty to be clear about the alcohol content so that the people we want to help can make an informed decision.

CHAPTER 7

HOW CAN I HELP OTHERS?

IMPROVING YOUR SELECTION SKILLS

If you want to help others with the remedies the first thing you need to do is to learn the remedies well This may sound obvious, but in fact most of us tend to learn best the four or five remedies that we use most often ourselves. Then when we start to help other people we are unconsciously looking for the slightest indications for these remedies, and often miss more obvious selections from among the 34 or so others that we don't usually use.

In my role as a teacher of this system I often see this in the classroom and in written work. One person sees Larch everywhere because that is the remedy she is taking, another feels himself surrounded by Vine types because that is what he himself needs to take.

So - how does one learn the remedies well? Reading this book is a help, obviously, but reading alone is not enough. You need to start to think with the remedies. Ideally the various categories, types and moods should be as familiar to you as the terms extrovert and introvert would be to a psychologist, or ego, id and super-ego to a psycho-analyst. You know the system really well when you are able to classify people under remedy headings in the same way that you can classify different shades of colour under main headings like red, green, blue, yellow and grey.

At the moment this may sound like a faint and far away ideal, but in fact you can get close to it surprisingly quickly if you take the trouble to build the remedies into your everyday life.

For example, you probably watch television drama from time to time. If you do you can't have failed to notice that the lives of most people in television drama are wholly out of balance, and that they spend every waking moment lurching from one crisis to another. Next time you are watching television you could amuse yourself by trying to pinpoint the type and mood remedies that the characters on the screen might need. Pay attention not just to what they say and the things they do, but look also at the way the actors use facial expression, body posture and mannerisms to communicate character. All of these things are simply exaggerated versions of the way we all communicate using a variety of different means, from words to body language to gesture.

You can do much the same thing with characters in films, plays and novels; with personalities from history; with people in the news; and with the people who you meet in everyday life. Most of our acquaintances are not quite so caricatured as the characters in soap operas, so this last may be slightly more difficult to do - but again the important thing is to get into the habit of thinking in terms of remedies. (And I am not suggesting that you attempt deep analysis of every acquaintance – simply notice the observations you would make anyway, and apply the system of 38 remedies to those observations.)

To avoid the trap of reading your own remedies into the people around you, refer frequently to the list of remedy indications and try to be more exact in your choice. Is so-and-so really Centaury, as your intuition tells you? Or would Wild Rose or Walnut be more appropriate? To decide, imagine the same person if she were an out-and-out Wild Rose or Walnut how close to the real person is your exaggerated Wild Rose?

If you are having trouble learning particular remedies, or remembering the differences between particular pairs of remedies (Larch and Elm, for example - which are both for 'lack of confidence' - or Gentian and Gorse, or Scleranthus and Wild Oat), then the same kind of technique can be used again. Just imagine a person in a situation, such as attending a job interview, and ask yourself how that person would react if he needed this or that remedy.

For example, in a Larch state the interviewee would be convinced that he was going to fail. He might not try very hard for this reason, and might even decide not to bother to turn up at all. In an Elm state the same person would be quite capable of doing the job and deep down would know his own abilities. He would go to the interview - but on hearing the extent of the responsibilities that go with the job he would become concerned about whether he could take them on in addition to all the other things that he is already committed to. His would be a crisis of confidence caused by the prospect of additional responsibilities. The Larch reaction would be a chronic lack of confidence that causes him to avoid taking responsibility in the first place.

Imagining people in situations like this is an excellent way to improve your knowledge of what the remedies are for, and so get to know the 38 remedies on a more intimate level. When you come to try to select remedies for other people the insight gained in these games will prove invaluable.

FAMILY AND FRIENDS

This book cannot teach you how to be a practitioner. Nevertheless, some of the skills that a practitioner calls on can be very useful when you are trying to help someone to select remedies. Here are a few basic tips:

Firstly, remember to listen to what is being said. This should be obvious, but many of us find it difficult to really listen to what someone else is saying. Instead we may be busy thinking about what we are going to say next, or thinking about how we felt when the same thing happened to us last year. Knowing the remedies really well is one way of helping yourself to listen: if you are trying to work out the subtle difference between Gentian and Gorse while your friend is telling you about her depression, you are probably going to miss the clues that indicate a different remedy entirely.

A related point is to remember why you are listening. If you become too interested in the story your friend is telling you might lose sight of the fact that you should be trying to work out how the story affected her, and not wondering how it is going to end. Secondly, don't be afraid to leave a silence. If your friend stops talking for a moment but is obviously collecting her thoughts you don't need to jump straight in with a question. It can be better to wait and allow her the time she needs to work things out in her mind.

Thirdly, if you do ask questions, try not to direct your friend towards the answers you want. For example, you might feel that she looks tired and so may need either Hornbeam or Olive. If you ask questions like: 'Are you tired first thing in the morning or last thing at night?' or 'Do you get tired at the end of the day?' you are not leaving her any room to talk about how she actually feels, and it is no surprise that you will get confirmation of your selection, and give her either Hornbeam or Olive.

It is better, then to ask open questions - in other words, questions that cannot be answered with a 'yes' or 'no', and do not restrict the range of possible answers. Open questions tend to begin with the words 'what', 'when', 'who' or 'how'. So better questions for your tired-looking friend might be 'What sort of things make you feel tired?', 'When do you get tired?', or 'How do you feel right now?' Each of these gives her space to choose her own response.

Fourthly, try to share your knowledge of the remedies so as to involve your friend in the selection process. Asking open questions goes some way towards achieving this, but you can go further still by explaining which remedies you are considering, and telling your friend what they are for. That way she has an opportunity to learn some of the remedy indications herself and can decide for herself which of two possible remedies is closest to how she feels. She can also disagree with your choice of remedies if she feels that you have got it wrong.

Sometimes we may be reluctant to do this. It can be particularly awkward if we are thinking about remedies whose indications are less than flattering. Few of us would mind hearing that Larch and White Chestnut mean we are a bit lacking in confidence and inclined to worry too much - but how would we feel knowing that Heather, Willow and Beech mean that we are considered to be self-pitying, intolerant bores ...

At the risk of making an understatement, explaining the remedies calls for more than a little tact. Perhaps the first thing to stress is that all the remedy states are normal, everyday human emotions, and that all of us feel these things from time to time. Following on from this you could explain the need for Willow by giving an example of when you had to use it and why. (Keep your example short, however - you don't want to hog the stage and stop your friend from telling you the things you need to know.)

Then you can relate the choice of remedies back to the things that your friend has said during the conversation. For example, she might have mentioned that her husband is getting on her nerves; you could remind her of this and say that Beech is the remedy to help us to get our tolerance back so that we can deal better with things that annoy us.

Finally, you can stress the positive aspect of the remedies - and if you look back through the remedy indications in chapter 4 you will see that every remedy does indeed have a positive aspect. You could for example explain the selection of Heather by stressing the fact that it will help your friend to look beyond her immediate concerns so that she can get her problems back into perspective. That way they will not bother her so much and she will be able to relate better to other people.

If you try to follow these basic rules and apply in addition a little common sense you will be able to help lots of people with the remedies. And once the word gets out that you have helped one of your friends or relations in this way, don't be surprised when more requests for help come your way.

SELECTING FOR YOUNGER CHILDREN

Some people find it difficult to select remedies for younger children. In many ways this is a pity because children actually respond very quickly to the remedies. Perhaps this is because their true feelings are closer to the surface and they haven't yet learned to conceal what they feel from the outside world, and from themselves.

It is in fact quite easy to select remedies for children, even when they are too young to explain how they feel. One can even select for babies who can barely communicate at all.

The key to doing this is of course observation and empathy.

Spend some time with the child while he is playing, and look at how he reacts. Is he short tempered or patient? Does he like to spend a long time absorbed in one activity or does he go from one thing to another? If he falls over or hurts himself, how does he behave? Putting these clues together you can soon come up with a mix of remedies - and because the remedies are harmless there is no danger involved if you have selected the wrong ones. All that will happen if you get it wrong is that the mix will have no effect.

Some remedies are certainly more used than others for small children. Rescue Remedy is a favourite, because it is always near at hand for accidents and upsets. Walnut is another useful remedy to keep in the nursery. It can be given to help children get used to the various stages that they go through in the early years, from being born, to getting teeth, to weaning, to starting school. And for the inevitable temper tantrums you could try Cherry Plum, to help junior stay in control of his own scary emotions.

The dosage for children is the same as for adults. For very small babies four drops from the treatment bottle can be added to a milk feed. If the mother takes the drops herself the effects will pass after a time to the baby through the breast milk. For older children you can mix the drops in with food or fruit juice.

A PRACTITIONER'S STORY

'Louise, William's mother, phoned me for an appointment. She said she got my telephone number from another mum she met at the baby clinic. Her Doctor was against complementary therapies and referred to them as "mumbo-jumbo" and "a load of rubbish", but she said she was so desperate she would try anything.

'I could hear William screaming as I parked my car and walked up the path to the front door. Louise looked totally exhausted - eyes red with dark rings underneath, very pale, hair not brushed, and wearing a dressing-gown (it was 2 pm). She apologised for the untidy state of the house and offered me a cup of tea, saying she hadn't had a chance to make one for herself that day. I accepted and held William while she made it.

William continued to scream very loudly. He was rigid and stiff and made constant, jerky movements with his arms, legs and head. He seemed very hot and looked very red.

'I introduced Louise to the remedies, and explained their gentle and benign action. Conversation was very difficult due to William's screaming, interspersed with little coughs, but I asked Louise about her pregnancy.

'She had gone through a difficult time, always throwing up, and had spent the second and third months in bed as a miscarriage was feared. The hospital had assured her that William had been unaffected by all this. When asked, she said that William had kicked and moved around a lot "almost as if he couldn't wait to get out and get on with it".

The birth had been straightforward but Louise said that William began to splutter, cry and yell almost immediately, and could not be pacified. He kept the whole maternity wing awake until a private room was made available. Louise chose to bottle-feed William and found he was very difficult to feed as he just took gulps in between screams and coughed most of it up again. It all took a long time and he was slightly underweight.

'I asked Louise about the rest of the family. She already had one daughter and had no problems with her as a baby. Her daughter had not taken to William as the crying and screaming kept her awake at night (she was falling asleep at school). He'd disrupted everything and didn't want to be cuddled or loved. Her partner worked long hours to make ends meet, and couldn't stand William's constant
screaming. He had gone to stay with his mother and only returned for clean clothes.

'Throughout our conversation William continued to scream loudly except for two occasions when, utterly exhausted, he fell into a brief and fitful sleep, in which he twitched, moved and whimpered. Almost as soon as he dozed off he coughed, which woke him up, and the screaming began again. Louise said that the longest span he'd slept since birth was one hour and thirty five minutes. He could not be pacified or comforted, remained very stiff (while asleep as well as awake) and I felt he would prefer to be left alone rather than be held or fussed. Louise confirmed this.

'The cough was not dry, but sounded like mucus in the throat, not on the chest. It had been there since birth. Her GP said it was due to his not having his airways sucked out properly in the delivery room, and said he would probably grow out of it at around age six months. If he didn't something would then be done.

'Louise told me that she was unable to go out at all as people stared at William. She relied on her daughter for shopping, and no-one was willing to baby-sit for William. Neighbours had complained about the noise.

'I considered which remedies were required. I decided on Crab Apple for its cleansing properties, Olive for his total exhaustion, Impatiens for his irritation and his wanting to be left alone, and Cherry Plum for his loss of control - he seemed at the end of his tether.

'Other remedies that crossed my mind - but which I decided against - were Vervain (the fretting was not of this nature), Water Violet (there was a need to be left alone, but this was more Impatiens in nature), Rock Water (there was physical rigidity, but it was more connected with Impatiens and Cherry Plum), Star of Bethlehem (there were no known shocks or birth traumas) and Walnut (I felt his adjustment to life was not a major consideration). 'I felt Impatiens could be his type remedy, as it was indicated even before birth.

'I explained all the chosen remedies to Louise and she agreed with all the indications except she was convinced that the crab apples in their garden were poisonous. I did my best to convince her otherwise but she phoned her father to check. The father confirmed that crab apples were quite safe - but then began to shout at her for having some quack in the house and told her not to let me anywhere near the baby. I could hear this from across the room.

'I gave William back to Louise so I could mix up the remedies. I explained the dose and that it should be administered in a little cooled, boiled water. While I did this Louise changed William and tried to feed him. There was no change in his behaviour. I made sure that Louise still had my telephone number, emphasised again the benign action of the remedies, and tried to give Louise reassurance, and to instil hope and confidence in the remedies.(William continued to scream.)

'I felt I'd built up a reasonable rapport, considering that Louise was very wary and suspicious - even a little hostile - at first. I left after one and a half hours feeling I needed some Rescue Remedy and a lie down in a darkened room. I could still hear William screaming as I got into my car. 'When I arrived home about three quarters of an hour later there was a hysterical message on my phone from Louise, wanting me to call back at once. William was very ill! What had I done to him!?

'I phoned straight back. Louise had given William his first dose, and he'd stopped crying almost immediately and fallen asleep. I explained that this was the best we could hope for, tried to calm her, explained again that the remedies are totally harmless. Louise was still very upset and angry, convinced I'd poisoned her baby.

'A few days later Louise phoned again. After her last call to me, she bundled William into a blanket and ran with him to her GP's surgery. A locum doctor had assured her that William was just sleeping, albeit very deeply. He encouraged her to continue with the remedies as all else had failed. William slept until 10 pm, when Louise woke him to be fed. She gave him a second dose of remedies at the same time; he cried a little but was soon asleep again. He slept until 2 am, when Louise panicked and woke him once more. He coughed a little but didn't cry. She was so worried she called her GP's number and the locum doctor visited at around 3 am. He was quite cross and said, again, that William was absolutely OK. Not convinced, an hour later she carried William to the casualty department at the local hospital, where he was pronounced to be fine. One of the nurses there said that she used the remedies and Louise was very much reassured by this and decided to continue with William's treatment.

'During the ensuing week, William's cough had steadily improved and was now gone. He had settled into a routine, sleeping twelve hours each night, and being woken at 10 pm to be fed. He was now feeding well. Sometimes he cried a little but the screaming had stopped completely, and he slept peacefully without jerking or being rigid. Louise's partner had moved back, a neighbour had offered to baby-sit from time to time and her daughter had brought a school friend to meet William.

'When I visited by appointment a few weeks later I was amazed at the change in William, and absolutely thrilled to see him so calm and content. His remedies were used up and Louise asked for some more. I felt that the Crab Apple, Cherry Plum and Olive were no longer required, but I put a couple of drops of Impatiens into a treatment bottle as I felt it might be a good idea to continue with his type remedy for a little longer. A couple of weeks later, when the bottle ran out, I said I felt he didn't need the remedies any more, that they had done their work. Louise got very agitated, worried that William's problems would return. After much reassurance from me that everything would be fine, and that she could always call me if it wasn't, she agreed to see how William got on without the remedies.

'Over the next couple of months several of Louise's friends contacted me, having been referred by her, and when I next bumped into her and the rest of the family it was at the railway station. They had just returned from a weekend away and William had coped with a long, crowded train journey with no problems. He still slept well, the cough hadn't returned, and he remained relaxed and well balanced.

'I was quite surprised at how quickly William returned from such an extreme state to a state of equilibrium. Now I have had more experience with babies I know that they do seem to respond very quickly. It was a great privilege to work with William and I can't help smiling every time I think of the brilliant outcome thanks to Dr Bach's remedies.'

HELPING ANIMALS

The problems involved in selecting for small children are of course magnified when trying to select for animals. This is probably why people turn to Rescue Remedy so much, and to the other remedies so little. Yet given a little thought and study it is perfectly possible to make a more focused selection of remedies.

You need to start by considering what life looks like to the species you are dealing with. Every species sees things differently from us, and also differently from each other, and you need to attempt to understand what the differences are.

We could take dogs as an example. Dogs are pack animals. In the wild they will usually live and hunt in a group. In captivity they see their human family as the pack. They are hierarchical animals and not democratic. In other words the strongest and most capable animal in a group will be the pack leader, and the question of who is dominant between two animals is one that has to be decided before normal doggy relations can be established. In a human family the dog needs to know its place, and that place should be clearly defined as the bottom of the family pecking order. If the dog comes anywhere else it can lead to problems.

Knowing a bit about dogs helps you to see how you might be causing problems rather than providing the solution. For example, if you have two dogs and one is bullying the other, do you make a fuss of the underdog? - It might appear like the natural thing to do, but as pack leader you are in effect singling out the subservient dog and promoting it above its superior. The dominant dog may well try more bullying in order to re-establish its position.

The answer in this case would be to make more of a fuss of the dominant animal. This can be done in small ways, such as giving it the first food bowl and saying hello to it before you say hello to the other one. This alone can be enough to resolve the problem.

Dominance games can take place between dogs and humans because to the dog both are in the same pack. The world of the rabbit is very different.

A rabbit is a prey animal, and in the wild being picked up by a large predator like a human being would be the last thing the rabbit would experience before being eaten. So while Vine may have a place in treating dominant dogs, it would almost certainly be a mistake to select Vine for a rabbit that has just bitten you. Fear remedies like Mimulus and Rock Rose are far more likely to be useful.

If you do a bit of reading about the natural history of the species you are treating you can go a long way towards understanding the mental world view of that species. Look in particular for information on social habits (are they herd animals or loners?), feeding habits (do they hunt or are they hunted?) and sex differences (how do males and females behave?).

But this is just the start, because even when treating animals you must still aim to make selections for individuals rather than the whole species. Knowing about the latter gives you a feel for what is most likely in terms of responses to particular problems. However, individual reactions still depend on the individual personality of the individual animal.

It is easier by far to select remedies for an animal that lives with us as one of the family. Most of us know the personalities of the animals in our home almost as well as we know those of our human companions. It is obviously more difficult when the animal concerned is not one you know well - such as sheep number 38 out of 250, or the stray cat in the street.

Nevertheless, even in this situation it is possible to go quite a long way. Look at the animal, and ask yourself how it compares with the average for its species. Is it particularly curious (for a sheep); or surprisingly keen to make friends (for a cat)? Are there any unusual behavioural quirks that make it stand out from the crowd? If it is under stress for some reason, how does it seem to go about coping with that stress?

Looking for these kinds of things will give you a sketch of the individual animal. Once you relate this back to the remedies you should be able to come up with a number of possible remedies that may be appropriate. At that point it is simply a question of choosing those that seem most appropriate. And remember that the remedies are entirely safe and cannot do any harm - a comfort when you are forced by necessity to rely on a certain amount of educated guesswork.

DOSAGE FOR ANIMALS

Once you have made a selection you need to find a way to give the remedies to the animal. In fact dosage for all animals is the same as it is for humans, regardless of size and weight. That is to say, four drops four times a day from a made-up treatment bottle - and you can in fact give drops from a treatment bottle, either direct (making sure that the animal doesn't swallow or bite the glass dropper) or via a sugar lump or some other favourite treat.

However, it can be more convenient to use other methods. You can add the remedies to a water bowl or bucket, or to food, and they will have the same effect. Many people rub the drops onto ears or paws, either so that the animal will take in the effects via the bloodstream, or knowing that it will lick off the drops (cats will do this almost without fail).

The important rule if you want to give the remedies like this is to use enough remedy. You want to be sure that however little the animal drinks it will be getting at least the equivalent of four drops from a treatment bottle. If you are making up a bowl of water for a dog then two drops of each individual remedy (four of Rescue Remedy) will be sufficient. In effect this is the same as making up a glass of water for a human being. But if the animal is larger, such as a horse or cow, and so is drinking from a much larger vessel, then you will have to add more of each remedy. The rule of thumb is to slightly more than double the dose: five drops of individual remedies, ten drops of Rescue Remedy.

It doesn't matter if two or more animals share a dosed water bowl, since the animals that do not need the remedies will not be affected by them. Of course, if two animals are both being treated using different remedies then you will have to find a way of dosing them separately.

EASTER BUNNIES

This story comes from Lucille Arcouet, a Bach practitioner in New York:

'Just after Easter I was in a local hardware store and saw a cage with two rabbits in it. They were left over from the holiday, and nobody wanted them, so I took them home with me.

'I hadn't thought about my two dogs - West Highland Terriers - and what their reaction would be to the new arrivals - Westies are hunters by instinct, so what they saw was something to chase and eat.

'I immediately made up a mix for the dogs. I put in Chicory for selfish possessiveness (the dogs love sitting on my lap and did not like having to share), Walnut to help them get used to the change, Holly for their jealousy, Cherry Plum to help them keep their self control, and Willow for resentment.

'They responded very quickly. Within three days the dogs and rabbits had bonded and were bounding about the living room together, nuzzling each other happily. Now if I say to the dogs "Where are your bunnies?" they will run to wherever the rabbits are.'

LEGAL CONSIDERATIONS WHEN HELPING ANIMALS

In some parts of the world there are strict laws governing who can and who cannot treat animals. In the United Kingdom, for example, it is illegal to treat any animal that belongs to someone else unless a qualified veterinary surgeon has referred the animal to you. You can treat your own animals, and give emergency help to save a life, but that's all. Similar laws are in force in many states in the United States of America.

If you are not sure about the legal position where you live then you need to seek advice before you offer help to someone else's animal.

TREATING PLANTS

The remedies can work just as well for plants as they do for people and animals. A man going into hospital, a dog suffering an illness and a plant infested with parasites are all under stress. So it is no surprise that the remedies can help all three of them.

The difficulty with plants is of course selecting appropriate remedies. For this reason the obvious remedies are the most often used: Rescue Remedy for any stressful event or illness; Crab Apple for attacks by fungus or insects; and Walnut to help the plant to adjust after re-potting or transplantation to a new garden.

It is possible to go further, although more difficult. You can start by looking at the shape of the plant and the way it is holding itself. A drooping plant might need Willow, or Gentian, or Gorse, or Olive, while a plant that seems to resist everything and go on blooming might benefit from Oak or Agrirnony. And you can try to put yourself in the plant's position and select remedies based on how you think you would feel in that position.

There will always be guesswork involved, of course, but because the remedies cannot do any harm you can experiment a little without worrying about the consequences.

The dosage for plants is once again as for humans. As long as the plant will get all the remedy you can make up a treatment bottle in the normal way, dropping the four drop dose into the middle of the plant four times a day.

You may find it more convenient to give the remedies using a watering can or sprayer. To water a single plant add two drops of each remedy (four of Rescue) to a little water in the can, or in a sprayer. If you are watering a larger area then add about five drops of each single remedy, or ten drops of Rescue Remedy, to each can full of water.

You would use the same strength of remedy in the watering can if you were giving remedies to a tree. The trick here is to water the ground that is sheltered by the branches. The roots of the tree will cover roughly the same area, so that the remedy will get to them most effectively.

The remedy stays in the soil along with the water and is absorbed gradually by the root system. This means that there is no need to water more than usual. However, if you are giving drops from a treatment bottle you will need to repeat the dose - at least four times a day.

CHAPTER 8

WHAT DO I DO IF....

I GET STUCK?

GETTING HELP AND ADVICE

Or Bach's aim was to create a simple system that anyone could use. 'It requires no science,' he once said, 'only a little knowledge and sympathy and understanding of human nature.'

Nevertheless, we all have times when our problems weigh us down, or seem so complicated that we need some help seeing past them and actually selecting the remedies we need. This is when it is useful to be able to get help and advice on the remedies.

The Dr Edward Bach Centre has always performed this role, and continues to do so today. It offers a free service. You can contact the Bach Centre by letter, phone, fax or email and receive advice to help you see your way forward.

Of course, some problems are too complex to be resolved over the phone or in writing, and that is when it can be helpful to go to see someone face to face. That is the time to think about going to see a qualified practitioner.

HOW DO I FIND A PRACTITIONER?

In many parts of the world it is possible for anyone to set up as a practitioner or therapist. The inevitable result is that there are people working in complementary medicine who are not well suited to that profession. Bach Flower Remedies are no exception, and as a potential client you will want to ensure that you are going to receive a good service. How then do you go about finding a competent practitioner?

One way is to contact the Bach Centre to see if there is a registered practitioner near you. Practitioners registered with the Dr Edward Bach Foundation, which is the Bach Centre's registering body, have all gone through an approved training course that includes classroom teaching and set written work studies, and every practitioner registered with the Foundation has agreed to abide by a strict Code of Practice that has been written to enforce acceptable standards of professional behaviour.

If there isn't a registered practitioner nearby then you may still be able to find a competent person if you approach the main national distributor for the remedies in the country where you live. They will often have details of local practitioners that they can pass on.

Failing that you can ask at your local health food shop or pharmacy to see if they can suggest a reliable person. Often this is the best option, because the local shop will tend to know local practitioners very well, and will be able to give you some informal advice on the person who will be best suited for you.

CONTACTING A PRACTITIONER

When you contact a practitioner for the first time there are a few questions you should ask so as to be sure that you know what kind of service you will receive. For example:

• How much will the consultation cost? What exactly does the charge include? Most practitioners will make an hourly charge that will include a mixed treatment bottle, and you need to be happy with the cost before you go ahead.

• Does the practitioner use genuine Bach Flower Remedies? There are many other flower essences on the market nowadays. Most are not licensed, and not all of them are made using the right plants or the right methods. You need to be happy with the quality of the medicines that you will be asked to take.

• How will remedies be selected? Practitioners registered with the Dr Edward Bach Foundation use the simple consultation interview to select remedies, and this has been found to be the most reliable method. Some practitioners select remedies using muscle testing, dowsing or other more occult techniques, and in this context these techniques can be highly subjective and misleading.

• Does the practitioner adhere to any code of practice, ethics or conduct, or belong to any professional body? How would you go about making a complaint if you felt you had not been treated properly? You can write to the Dr Edward Bach Foundation if you feel that a registered Bach practitioner has behaved in an unprofessional way, and the Foundation will investigate breaches of the Code. You need to be equally sure of the complaints procedure if you are using a non-registered practitioner.

There are many very good practitioners around, and not all of them are registered with the Foundation. And of course if you feel that you want to see someone who uses muscle testing or works with other essences then that is entirely your choice. The important thing is to be aware of what is being offered to you so that you can make an informed choice.

WHAT HAPPENS DURING A CONSULTATION?

A consultation should be a straightforward affair, and reflect the simplicity of the therapy itself. The practitioner will start by asking you how much you know about the remedies, and will tell you a little about the system if that seems appropriate. Then she will ask why you have come and what you are having trouble with. The aim will be to find out how you feel about your current situation, and as far as possible the practitioner will avoid putting words into your mouth so that you can say for yourself how you feel.

There is no reason to fear the consultation or to be embarrassed at talking about your emotions. All the remedies reflect normal human emotions, and the practitioner will have gone through all possible negative emotions at some time or other just like all of us have. Nevertheless, if you do feel that you need some Rescue Remedy or Mimulus at the start to settle you down then just ask the practitioner, who will be only too happy to oblige.

The practitioner will aim to listen more than she talks, and if she does ask questions they will be aimed at finding out what depression or unhappiness or stress actually feels like to you. She may ask about your reactions to particular situations, or even to hypothetical situations, in order to ascertain what might be your type remedy.

Most first consultations last about an hour. Towards the end of this time the practitioner will sum up for you what she has understood, giving you a chance to correct any misunderstandings. She will then go through the remedies she thinks might apply, explaining to you her reasons for each selection. This too gives you an opportunity to say if you do not agree with a particular choice.

Finally, she will mix up a treatment bottle for you, or perhaps help you to do this yourself or give you the address of a pharmacy that will mix up the bottle for you.

Arrangements for a follow-up appointment might be made there and then, or you might be invited to phone in to make a further appointment when you need to. Most follow-up visits will be arranged for two or three weeks after the first consultation, as this is the time that the treatment bottle will last.

HOW MANY CONSULTATIONS WILL I NEED?

There is no hard and fast rule about how many consultations you will need to help get things moving for you. Certainly good practitioners will be keen to see you starting to select remedies for yourself as soon as you feel able to do this. They will be aware that this is a self-help therapy, and will want to encourage you to use it in this way rather than building up dependency on a practitioner. This is why we often say at the Bach Centre that the best practitioners are the ones who lose all their clients, and are happy to do so.

Printed in Great Britain
by Amazon

87759341R00078